Instructor's Resource Manual for
MATERNAL & CHILD NURSING CARE

INSTRUCTOR'S RESOURCE MANUAL FOR

MATERNAL & CHILD NURSING CARE

THIRD EDITION

MARCIA L. LONDON, RN, MSN, APRN, CNS, NNP-BC
Senior Clinical Instructor and Ret. Director of Neonatal
Nurse Practitioner Program
Beth-El College of Nursing and Health Sciences
University of Colorado, Colorado Springs, Colorado
Staff Clinical Nurse
Urgent Care and After Hours Clinic
Colorado Springs, Colorado

PATRICIA A. WIELAND LADEWIG, PhD, RN
Professor and Academic Dean
Rueckert-Hartman College for Health Professions
Regis University
Denver, Colorado

JANE W. BALL, RN, CPNP, DrPH
Consultant
American College of Surgeons
Gaithersburg, Maryland

RUTH C. MCGILLIS BINDLER, RNC, PhD
Professor
Washington State University
College of Nursing
Spokane, Washington

KAY J. COWEN, RNC, MSN
Clinical Associate Professor
University of North Carolina at Greensboro
Greensboro, North Carolina

Contributors
Michael D. Aldridge, MSN, RN, CCRN, CNS
University of Texas at Austin

Jenny C. Clapp, RN, MSN
University of North Carolina Greensboro School of Nursing

Bernadette Dragich, PhD, APRN, BC
Bluefield State College, West Virginia

Pearson
Boston   Columbus   Indianapolis   New York   San Francisco   Upper Saddle River
Amsterdam   Cape Town   Dubai   London   Madrid   Milan   Munich   Paris   Montreal   Toronto
Delhi   Mexico City   Sao Paulo   Sydney   Hong Kong   Seoul   Singapore   Taipei   Tokyo

Notice: Care has been taken to confirm the accuracy of information presented in this book. The authors, editors, and the publisher, however, cannot accept any responsibility for errors or omissions or for consequences from application of the information in this book and make no warranty, express or implied, with respect to its contents.

The authors and publisher have exerted every effort to ensure that drug selections and dosages set forth in this text are in accord with current recommendations and practice at time of publication. However, in view of ongoing research, changes in government regulations, and the constant flow of information relating to drug therapy and reactions, the reader is urged to check the package inserts of all drugs for any change in indications or dosage and for added warning and precautions. This is particularly important when the recommended agent is a new and/or infrequently employed drug.

Publisher: Julie Levin Alexander
Assistant to Publisher: Regina Bruno
Editor-in-Chief: Maura Connor
Assistant to the Editor-in-Chief: Deirdre MacKnight
Executive Acquisitions Editor: Kim Mortimer
Assistant to the Executive Acquisitions Editor: Marion Gottlieb
Development Editor: Molly Ward
Director of Marketing: David Gesell
Marketing Coordinator: Michael Sirinides
Managing Editor, Production: Patrick Walsh
Production Editor: Lynn Steines, S4Carlisle Publishing Services
Production Liaison: Anne Garcia
Media Project Manager: Rachel Collett
Manufacturing Manager: Ilene Sanford
Senior Design Coordinator: Maria Guglielmo-Walsh
Cover Design: Wanda España
Composition: S4Carlisle Publishing Services
Printer/Binder: Bind-Rite Graphics / Robbinsville
Cover Printer: Bind-Rite Graphics / Robbinsville

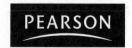

www.pearsonhighered.com

10 9 8 7 6 5 4 3 2 1
ISBN-13: 978-0-13-509720-5
ISBN-10:   0-13-509720-7

CONTENTS

PREFACE

As teachers involved in nursing education, you are participants in a rapidly changing environment. Limited clinical sites, nontraditional students with limited time for lengthy assignments, and changing student learning styles are just a few of the factors that demand a rethinking of how you go about the "business" of education. This *Instructor's Resource Manual*, written to accompany *Maternal & Child Nursing Care, Third Edition* by London, Ladewig, Ball, Bindler, and Cowan, is designed to assist you in providing an optimal learning experience for your students and their many learning needs.

Each chapter of the *Instructor's Resource Manual* is thoroughly integrated with the corresponding chapter in the main textbook. Chapters are organized by objectives, and the teaching unit flows from these objectives. You will find the following features to support the objectives:

- **Concepts for Lecture** in the manual may be used in their entirety for class presentation, or they may be merged with the classroom activities for a mixture of teaching styles that will meet the needs of students with various learning styles.

- **PowerPoints** contain the Concepts for Lecture along with selected figures, tables, and boxes from the textbook. These are available in PowerPoint on the companion website, *www.mynursingkit.com.*

- **Suggestions for Classroom and Clinical Activities** attempt to go beyond the traditional activities that have been the mainstay of maternal-newborn and pediatric nursing education for many years. These are designed to help you design appropriate exercises and applications in the classroom, in the skills laboratory, and in the clinical setting and make use of the many media assets and exercises available on the companion website, *www.mynursingkit.com.*

- **Media and visual assets** available for that chapter are also listed. These identify for you—the instructor—all the specific media resources and activities available for that chapter on *www.mynursingkit.com,* as well as all the images from the textbook that are included in the Image Bank PowerPoint presentation,

also on MyNursingKit.com. Chapter by chapter, the **media listings** help you decide what resources from the companion website to assign to enhance your course and your students' ability to apply concepts from the book into practice.

This Instructor's Resource Manual also contains a Strategies for Success module that includes discussion on learning theories, planning for instruction, how to use effective pedagogies, assessing learning, and more. There is also a guide on *Teaching Nursing to Students Who Speak English as a Non-native Language.* This tool is intended to guide you in reaching across cultural barriers to train nurses.

The following additional resources are also available to accompany this textbook. For more information or sample copies, please contact your Pearson sales representative or visit *www.mypearsonstore.com:*

- **MyNursingKit** (*www.mynursingkit.com*) This student and instructor resource gives you everything you need in one place! Students can use this site as an online study guide and source for additional resources. Instructors can find chapter specific Power-Point lecture notes, test item questions, and instructor manual materials.

- **Online Course Management Systems.** Instructor and student resources are available within our Course Compass platform. For more information on Course Compass and other course management systems such as Blackboard or WebCT, please contact your Pearson sales representative or visit *www.mypearsonstore.com.*

- **MyNursingLab.** A valuable tool for formative assessment and customized student remediation. This online tool gives students the opportunity to test themselves on key concepts and skills in pediatric nursing. By using MyNursingLab, students can track their own progress through the course and use customized, media-rich, study plan activities to help achieve success in the classroom, in clinical, and ultimately on the NCLEX-RN. MyNursingLab allows instructors to monitor class progress as students move through the curriculum.

TEACHING NURSING TO STUDENTS WHO SPEAK ENGLISH AS A NON-NATIVE LANGUAGE

We are fortunate to have so many multinational and multilingual nursing students in the United States in the 21st century. As our classrooms become more diverse, there are additional challenges to communication, but we in the nursing education community are ready. Our goal is to educate competent and caring nurses to serve the health needs of our diverse communities.

We know that ENNL students experience higher attrition rates than their native English-speaking counterparts. This is a complex problem. However, there are teaching strategies that have helped many students be successful.

The first step toward developing success strategies is understanding language proficiency. Language proficiency has four interdependent components. Each component is pertinent to nursing education. **Reading** is the first aspect of language. Any nursing student will tell you that there are volumes to read in nursing education. Even native speakers of English find the reading load heavy. People tend to read more slowly in their non-native language. They also tend to recall less. Non-native speakers often spend inordinate amounts of time on reading assignments. These students also tend to take longer to process exam questions.

Listening is the second component of language. Learning from lectures can be challenging. Some students are more proficient at reading English than at listening to it. It is not uncommon for ENNL students to understand medical terminology, but to become confused by social references, slang, or idiomatic expressions used in class. The spoken language of the teacher may be different in accent or even vocabulary from that experienced by immigrant students in their language education. ENNL students may not even hear certain sounds that are not present in their native languages. *Amoxicillin* and *Ampicillin*, for example, may sound the same. Asian languages do not have gender-specific personal pronouns (he, she, him, her, etc.). Asian students may become confused when the teacher is describing a case study involving people of different genders.

Speaking is the third component of language proficiency. People who speak with an accent are often self-conscious about it. They may hesitate to voice their questions or to engage in discussion. Vicious cycles of self-defeating behavior can occur in which a student hesitates to speak, resulting in decreased speaking skills, which results in more hesitation to speak. Students may develop sufficient anxiety about speaking that their academic outcomes are affected. Students tend to form study groups with others who have common first languages. Opportunities to practice English are therefore reduced, and communication errors are perpetuated. When the teacher divides students into small groups for projects, ENNL students often do not participate as much as others. If these students are anxious about speaking, they may withdraw from classroom participation. ENNL students may feel rejected by other students in a small group situation when their input is not sought or understood.

The fourth aspect of language is **writing**. Spelling and syntax errors are common when writing a non-native language. Teachers often respond to student writing assignments with feedback that is too vague to provide a basis for correction or improvement by ENNL students. When it comes to writing lecture notes, these students are at risk of missing important details because they may not pick up the teacher's cues about what is important. They might miss information when they spend extra time translating a word or concept to understand it, or they might just take more time to write what is being said.

Another major issue faced by ENNL nursing students is the culture of the learning environment. International students were often educated in settings where students took a passive role in the classroom. They may have learned that faculty are to be respected, not questioned. Memorization of facts may have been emphasized. It may be a shock to them when the nursing faculty expect assertive students who ask questions and think critically. These expectations cannot be achieved unless students understand them.

Finally, the European American culture, which forms the context for nursing practice, creates challenges. Because they are immersed in Euro-American culture and the culture of nursing, faculty may not see the potential sources of misunderstanding. For example, if a teacher writes a test question about what foods are allowed on a soft diet, a student who understands therapeutic diets may miss the question if he or she does not recognize the names of the food choices. Nursing issues with especially high culture connection are: food, behavior, law, ethics, parenting, games, or choosing the right thing to say. These topics are well represented in psychiatric nursing, which makes it a difficult subject for ENNL students.

MINIMIZING CULTURE BIAS ON NURSING EXAMS

Our goal is not really to eliminate culture from nursing or from nursing education. Nursing exists in a culture-dependent context. Our goal is to practice transcultural nursing and to teach nursing without undue culture bias.

Sometimes our nursing exam questions will relate to culture-based expectations for nursing action. The way to make these questions fair is to teach transcultural nursing and to clarify the cultural expectations of a nursing student in the Euro-American-dominated health care system. Students must learn the cultural aspects of the profession before they can practice appropriately within it. Like other cultures, the professional culture of nursing has its own language (medical terminology and nursing diagnoses, of course). We have our own accepted way of dress, our own implements, skills, taboos, celebrations, and behavior. The values accepted by our culture are delineated in the ANA Code of Ethics, and are passed down to our young during nursing education.

It is usually clear to nursing educators that students are not initially aware of all the aspects of the professional culture, and that these must be taught. The social context of nursing seems more obvious to educators, and is often overlooked in nursing education. Some aspects of the social context of nursing were mentioned previously (food, games, social activities, relationships, behavior, what to say in certain situations). Students must also learn these social behaviors and attitudes if they are to function fully in nursing. If they do not already know about American hospital foods, what to say when someone dies, how to communicate with an authority figure, or what game to play with a 5-year-old child, they must learn these things in nursing school.

Try for yourself the following test. It was written without teaching you the cultural expectations first.

CULTURE BIASED TEST

1. Following radiation therapy, an African American client has been told to avoid using her usual hair-care product due to its petroleum content. Which product should the nurse recommend that she use instead?
   a. Royal Crown hair treatment
   b. Dax Wave and Curl
   c. Long Aid Curl Activator Gel
   d. Wave Pomade

2. A Jewish client is hospitalized for pregnancy-induced hypertension during Yom Kippur. How should the nurse help this client meet her religious needs based on the tradition of this holy day?
   a. Order meals without meat/milk combinations.
   b. Ask a family member to bring a serving of *Marror* for the client.
   c. Encourage her to fast from sunrise to sunset.
   d. Remind her that she is exempt from fasting.

3. Based on the Puerto Rican concept of *compadrazco*, who is considered part of the immediate family and responsible for care of children?
   a. Parents, grandparents, aunts, uncles, cousins, and godparents
   b. Mother and father, older siblings
   c. Mother, father, any blood relative
   d. Parents and chosen friends (*compadres*) who are given the honor of childcare responsibility

4. A 60-year-old Vietnamese immigrant client on a general diet is awake at 11 PM on a summer night. What is the best choice of food for the nurse to offer to this client?
   a. warm milk
   b. hot tea
   c. ice cream
   d. iced tea

5. Which of the following positions is contraindicated for a client recovering from a total hip replacement?
   a. side-lying using an abductor pillow
   b. standing
   c. walking to the restroom using a walker
   d. sitting in a low recliner

When you took this test, did it seem unfair? It was intended to test nursing behaviors that were based on culture-specific situations. Your immigrant and ENNL students are likely to face questions like these on every exam.

Item 1 is about hair-care products for black hair. Option C is the only one that does not contain petroleum products. Students could know this, if they were given the information before the exam. Otherwise the item is culture-biased.

Item 2 is about the Jewish holiday Yom Kippur. To celebrate this holiday, it is customary to fast from sunrise to sunset, but people who are sick, such as the client in the question, are exempted from fasting. This question is only unfair if students did not have access to the information.

Item 3 expects you to know about *compadrazco*, in which parents, grandparents, aunts, uncles, cousins, and godparents are all considered immediate family. This can be an important point if you are responsible for visiting policies in a pediatrics unit.

Item 4 tests knowledge about the preferred drink for an immigrant Vietnamese client. Many people in Asia feel comforted by hot drinks and find cold drinks to be unsettling.

Item 5 does not seem so biased. If you understand total hip precautions, it is a pretty simple question, unless you have never heard of a "low recliner." An ENNL student who missed this question said, "I saw the chairs in clinical called 'geri chairs' and I know that the client cannot bend more than 90 degrees, but 'low recliner' was confusing to me. I imagined someone lying down (reclining) and I think this would not dislocate the prosthesis."

The best way to avoid culture bias on exams is to know what you are testing. It is acceptable to test about hip precautions, but not really fair to test about the names of furniture. The same is true of foods. Test about therapeutic diets, but not about the recipes (an African immigrant student advised us to say "egg-based food" instead of custard).

Behavior in social and professional situations is especially culture-bound. Behavior-based questions are common on nursing exams. Make behavior expectations explicit. Especially when a student is expected to act in a way that would be inappropriate in his or her social culture, these are very difficult questions. For example, we expect nurses to act assertively with physicians and clients. It is inappropriate for many Asian students to question their elders. When a client is their elder, these students will choose the option that preserves respect for the client over one that provides teaching. We must make our expectations very clear.

Finally, talk with your ENNL and immigrant students after your exams. They can provide a wealth of information about what confused them or what was ambiguous. Discuss your findings with your colleagues and improve your exams. Ultimately your exams will be clearer and more valid.

SUCCESS STRATEGIES

The following strategies were developed originally to help ENNL students. An interesting revelation is that they also help native English speakers who have learning styles that are not conducive to learning by lecture, or who read slowly, or have learning disabilities or other academic challenges.

STRATEGIES FOR PROMOTING ENNL STUDENT SUCCESS

1. You cannot decrease the reading assignments because some students read slowly, but you can help students prioritize the most important areas.
2. Allow adequate time for testing. The NCLEX® is not a 1-minute-per-question test anymore. Usually 1.5 hours is adequate for a 50-item multiple-choice exam.
3. Allow students to tape lectures if they want to. You might have lectures audiotaped and put in the library for student access.
4. Speak clearly. Mumbling and rapid, anxious speech are difficult to understand. If you have a problem with clarity, provide handouts containing the critical points. Provide the handouts anyway. You want to teach and test nursing knowledge, not note-taking skills.
5. Avoid slang and idiomatic expressions. This is harder than heck to do, but you can do it with practice. When you do use slang, explain it. This is especially important on exams. When in doubt about whether a word is confusing, think about what the dictionary definition would be; if there are two meanings, use another word.
6. Allow the use of translation dictionaries on exams. You can say that students must tell you what they are looking up, so they cannot find medical terminology that is part of the test.
7. Be aware of cultural issues when you are writing exams. Of course you will test on culture-specific issues, but be sure you are testing what you want to test (e.g., the student's knowledge of diets, not of recipes).
8. Feel free to use medical terminology, after all this is nursing school. However, when you use an important new term, write it on the board so students can spell it correctly in their notes.
9. In clinical, make the implied explicit. It seems obvious that safety is the priority, but if a student thinks the priority is respecting her elders, when a client with a new hip replacement demands to get out of bed there could be a disaster.
10. Hire a student who takes clear and accurate lecture notes to post his or her notes for use by ENNL and other students. The students will still attend class and take their own notes, but will have this resource to fill in the details that they miss.
11. SOA (spell out abbreviations).
12. Many international students learned to speak English in the British style. If something would be confusing to a British person, they will find it confusing.
13. Provide opportunities for students to discuss what they are learning with other students and faculty. A faculty member might hold a weekly discussion group where students bring questions. It can be interesting to find a student having no trouble tracing the path of a red cell from the heart to the portal vein, but having difficulty understanding what cream of wheat is ("I thought it was a stalk of grain in a bowl with cream poured on it").
14. Make it clear that questions are encouraged. When a student is not asking questions, and you think he or she may not understand, ask the student after class if he or she has questions. Make it easier for students to approach you by being approachable. Learn their names, and learn to pronounce them correctly. Hearing you try to pronounce their name might be humorous for them, and it will validate how difficult it is to speak other languages.
15. Take another look at basing grades on class participation. You may be putting inordinate demands on the ENNL students. Of course nurses must learn to work with others, but the nurse who talks most is not necessarily the best.
16. Be a role model for communication skills. You might even say in class when you talk about communication that if you respect a person who is trying to communicate with you, you will persist until you understand the message. Say, "Please repeat that," or "I think you said to put a chicken on my head, is that correct?" or "You want me to do what with the textbook?" It may be considered socially rude to ask people to repeat themselves repeatedly. Make it clear that this is not a social situation. In the professional role, we are responsible for effective communication. We cannot get away with smiling and nodding our heads.
17. In clinical, if a student has an accent that is difficult for the staff to understand, discuss clarification techniques (see 16 above) with the student and staff members. Make it explicit that it is acceptable for the student to ask questions and for the staff to ask for clarification.
18. If your college has a writing center where students can receive feedback on grammar and style before submitting papers, have students use it. If you are not so fortunate, view papers as a rough draft instead of a final product. Give specific feedback about what to correct and allow students to resubmit.
19. Make any services available to ENNL students available to all students (such as group discussions and notes). These services may meet the learning needs of many students while preventing the attitude that "they are different and they get something I don't."
20. Faculty attitudes are the most important determinant of a successful program to promote the success of ENNL nursing students. Talk with other faculty about the controversial issues. Create an organized program with a consistent approach among the faculty. The rewards will be well worth the work.

STRATEGIES FOR SUCCESS

Sandra DeYoung, Ed.D., R.N.

IMPROVING OUR TEACHING

Every faculty member wants to be a good teacher, and every teacher wants her or his students to learn. In particular, we want to achieve the student learning outcomes that our educational institutions say that we must achieve. How can we best meet both goals? We cannot just teach as we were taught. We have to learn a variety of teaching methods and investigate best practices in pedagogy. We also have to learn how to measure student learning outcomes in practical and efficient ways. The next few pages will introduce you to principles of good teaching and ways to evaluate learning. Keep in mind that this is only an introduction. For a more extensive study of these principles and pedagogies, you might consult the resources listed at the end of this introduction.

LEARNING THEORY

In order to improve our teaching, we must have some familiarity with learning theory. Nurses who come into educational roles without psychology of learning courses in their background should read at least an introductory-level book on learning theories. You should, for example, know something about stages and types of learning, how information is stored in memory and how it is retrieved, and how knowledge is transferred from one situation to another.

BEHAVIORIST THEORIES

Behaviorist theories are not in as much favor today as they were 25 years ago, but they still help to explain simple learning. Conditioning and reinforcement are concepts with which most educators are familiar. Conditioning explains how we learn some simple movements and behaviors that result in desired outcomes, such as a nurse responding when an alarm sounds on a ventilator. Reinforcement refers to the fact that behavior that is rewarded or reinforced tends to reoccur. Therefore, reinforcement is a powerful tool in the hands of an educator.

COGNITIVE LEARNING THEORIES

Cognitive learning theories are much more sophisticated and deal with how we process information by perceiving, remembering, and storing information. All of these processes are a part of learning. One of the most useful concepts in cognitive theory is that of mental schemata.

Schemata (plural) are units of knowledge that are stored in memory. For example, nurses must develop a schema related to aseptic technique. Once a schema is stored in memory, related information can be built on it. For instance, changing a dressing is easier to learn if the learner already has a schema for asepsis.

Metacognition is another concept identified in cognitive theories. This concept refers to thinking about one's thinking. To help learners who are having difficulty mastering certain material, you might ask them to think about how they learn best and to help them evaluate whether they really understand the material.

Transfer of learning occurs when a learner takes information from the situation in which it is learned and applies it to a new situation. Transfer is most likely to occur if the information was learned well in the first place, if it can be retrieved from memory, and if the new situation is similar to the original learning situation. Educators can teach for transfer by pointing out to students how a concept is applied in several situations so that learners know that the concept is not an isolated one, and the students begin to look for similar patterns in new situations.

ADULT LEARNING THEORIES

Adult learning theories help to explain how learning takes place differently for adults than for children. Adults usually need to know the practical applications for the information they are given. They also want to see how it fits with their life experiences. When teaching young adults and adults, nurse educators need to keep in mind adult motivation for learning.

LEARNING STYLE THEORIES

Learning style theories abound. Research has shown that some learners are visually oriented; some are more auditory or tactile learners; some are individualistic and learn best alone whereas others learn best by collaboration; some deal well with abstract concepts while others learn better with concrete information. Measurement instruments that can determine preferred learning styles are readily available. Although not many educators actually measure their students' learning styles, they should at least keep learning styles in mind when they plan their instruction.

PLANNING FOR INSTRUCTION

With some background knowledge of how students learn, the nurse educator can begin to plan the learning experiences. Planning includes developing objectives, selecting content, choosing pedagogies, selecting assignments, and planning for assessment of learning. All nurse educators come to the teaching process already knowing how to write objectives. Objectives can be written in the cognitive, psychomotor, and affective domains of learning. In the cognitive domain, they can be written at the knowledge, comprehension, application, analysis, and synthesis levels of complexity. The critical aspect of objectives is that you need to keep referring to them as you plan your lesson or course. They will help you focus on the "need to know" versus the "nice to know" material. They will help you decide on which assignments will be most suitable, and they will guide your development of evaluation tools.

SELECTING ASSIGNMENTS

Selecting and developing out-of-class assignments calls for creativity. You may use instructor manuals, such as this one, for ideas for assignments or you may also develop your own. To encourage learning through writing, you can assign short analysis papers, position papers, or clinical journals, all of which promote critical thinking. Nursing care plans of various lengths and complexity may be assigned. You may create reading guides with questions to help students read their textbooks analytically. You might also ask students to interview people or observe people to achieve various objectives.

USING EFFECTIVE PEDAGOGIES

Selecting teaching methods or pedagogies takes considerable time. You must consider what you are trying to achieve. To teach facts, you may choose to lecture or assign a computer tutorial. To change attitudes or motivate learners, you may use discussion, role-playing, or gaming. Developing critical thinking may be done effectively using critical thinking exercises, concept maps, group projects, or problem-based learning. There are what I will call *traditional* pedagogies, *activity-based* pedagogies, and *technology-based* pedagogies.

TRADITIONAL PEDAGOGIES

Traditional pedagogies include lecture, discussion, and questioning. Lecturing is an efficient way to convey a great deal of information to large groups of people. However, the lecture creates passive learning. Learners just sit and listen (or not) and do not interact with the information or the lecturer. Research has shown that students learn more from active learning techniques—that is, from being able to talk about, manipulate, reduce, or synthesize information. So, if you are going to lecture, it would be wise to intersperse lecture with discussion and questioning.

Discussion gives students an opportunity to analyze and think critically about information that they have read or were given in a lecture. By discussing key concepts and issues, they can learn the applicability of the concepts and see how they can transfer to varied situations. Discussions can be formal or informal, but they generally work best if they are planned. For a formal discussion, students must be held accountable for preparing for it. The teacher becomes a facilitator by giving an opening statement or question, guiding the discussion to keep it focused, giving everyone a chance to participate, and summarizing at the end.

Questioning is a skill that develops over time. The first principle to learn is that you have to give students time to answer. Most teachers wait only one second before either repeating the question or answering it themselves. You should wait at least three to five seconds before doing anything, to allow students time to think and prepare a thoughtful answer. Research has revealed that most instructor-posed questions are at a very low level (lower-order), eliciting recall of facts. But questioning can be used to develop critical thinking if it is planned. Higher-order questions are those that require students to interpret information, to apply it to different situations, to think about relationships between concepts, or to assess a situation. If you ask higher-order questions during your classes or clinical experiences, students will rise to the occasion and will be challenged to provide thoughtful answers.

ACTIVITY-BASED PEDAGOGIES

Activity-based teaching strategies include cooperative learning, simulations, games, problem-based learning, and self-learning modules, among others. Cooperative learning is an old pedagogy that has received more research support than any other method. This approach involves learners working together and being responsible for the learning of group members as well as their own learning. Cooperative learning groups can be informal, such as out-of-class study groups, or can be formally structured in-class groups. The groups may serve to solve problems, develop projects, or discuss previously taught content.

Simulations are exercises that can help students to learn in an environment that is low risk or risk free. Students can learn decision making, for example, in a setting where no one is hurt if the decision is the wrong one. Simulations in skills laboratories are frequently used to teach psychomotor skills. Simulations can be written (case studies), acted out (role-playing), computer-based (clinical decision-making scenarios), or complex, technology-based (active simulation mannequins).

Games can help motivate people to learn. Factual content that can be rather boring to learn, such as medical terminology, can be turned into word games such as crossword puzzles or word searches. More complex games can teach problem solving or can apply previously learned information; board games or simulation games can be used for these purposes.

Problem-based learning (PBL) provides students with real-life problems that they must research and analyze and then develop possible solutions for. PBL is a group activity. The instructor presents the students with a brief problem statement. The student groups make lists of what they know and don't know about the problem. They decide what information they must collect in order to further understand the problem. As they collect the information and analyze it, they further refine the problem and begin to investigate possible solutions. The educator serves as a facilitator and resource during the learning process and helps keep the group focused.

Self-learning modules are a means of self-paced learning. They can be used to teach segments of a course or an entire course or curriculum. Modules should be built around a single concept. For example, you might design a module for a skills lab based on aseptic technique; or you could develop a module for a classroom course around the concept of airway impairment. Each module contains components such as an introduction, instructions on how to use the module, objectives, a pretest, learning activities, and a posttest. Learning activities within a module should address various learning styles. You should try to include activities that appeal to visual learners and tactile learners, conceptual learners and abstract learners, and individual and collaborative learners, for example. Those activities could be readings, audiovisuals, computer programs, group discussion, or skills practice. The educator develops and tests the module and then acts as facilitator and evaluator as learners work through the module.

TECHNOLOGY-BASED PEDAGOGIES

Technology-based pedagogies include computer simulations and tutorials, internet use, and distance-learning applications. Computer simulations were discussed briefly in the previous section. They include decision-making software in which a clinical situation is enacted and students are asked to work through the nursing process to solve problems and achieve positive outcomes. They also include simulation games such as SimCity, which can be a useful tool in teaching community health principles. Computer tutorials are useful for individual remedial work such as medication calculations or practice in answering multiple-choice test questions.

The internet is a rich resource for classroom use and for out-of-class assignments. The World Wide Web contains hundreds of websites that can be accessed for health-related information. Students need to be taught how to evaluate the worth of these websites. The criteria they should apply to this evaluation include identifying the intended audience, the currency of the information, the author's credentials or the affiliated organization, and content accuracy. Students may not know how to identify online journal sources compared to other websites. It is worth spending time, therefore, teaching students how to use the Web before giving them assignments that include Web use. If your classroom is internet-access enabled, you can visually demonstrate how to identify and use appropriate websites. For example, if you want students to find relevant information for diabetic teaching, you can show them the differing value of information from official diabetes associations versus pharmaceutical sites versus chat rooms or public forums.

You may be using this instructor manual in a distance-learning course. Distance learning takes the forms of interactive television classes, Webcasting, or online courses. In any form of distance learning, students are learning via the technology, but they are also learning about technology and becoming familiar with several computer applications. Those applications may include synchronous and asynchronous applications, streaming video, and multimedia functions.

ASSESSING LEARNING

You can assess or evaluate learning in a number of ways. Your first decision is whether you are just trying to get informal, ungraded feedback on how well students are learning in your class, or whether you are evaluating the students for the purpose of assigning a grade. Following are a number of techniques that can be used for one or both purposes.

CLASSROOM ASSESSMENT TECHNIQUES

Classroom assessment techniques (CATs) are short, quick, ungraded, in-class assessments used to gauge students' learning during or at the end of class. Getting frequent feedback on students' understanding helps educators to know if they are on the right track and if students are benefiting from the planned instruction. If you wait until you give a formal quiz or examination, you may have waited too long to help some students who are struggling with the material. The most popular CAT is probably the *minute paper*. This technique involves asking students to write down, in one or two minutes, usually at the end of class, the most important thing they learned that day or points that remain unclear. A related technique is the *muddiest point,* in which you ask the class to write down what the "muddiest" part of the class was for them. In nursing, *application cards* can be especially useful. After teaching about a particular concept or body of knowledge, and before you talk about the applications of the information, ask the students to fill out an index card with one possible clinical application of the information. This technique fosters application and critical thinking. Always leave class time during the following session to give feedback on the CAT results.

TESTS AND EXAMINATIONS

Tests and examinations are also used to assess or evaluate learning. Tests should be planned carefully to measure whether learning objectives have been met. You should form a test plan in which you decide the number of test items to include for each objective as well as the complexity of the items. Just as objectives can be written at the knowledge through synthesis levels of knowing, test items can be written at each level, too. Some types of items lend themselves to the lower levels of knowing, such as true-false and matching items, while multiple-choice and essay questions can be used to test higher levels.

TRUE-FALSE QUESTIONS

True-false questions are used simply to assess whether the student can determine the correctness of a fact or principle. This type of question should be used sparingly, because the student has a 50% chance of guessing the correct answer. Well-written true-false questions are clear and unambiguous. The entire statement should be totally true or totally false. An example of a question that is ambiguous is:

(T F) A routine urinanalyis specimen must be collected with clean technique and contain at least 100 ml.

The answer to this question is false because the specimen does not require 100 mL of volume. However, the clean technique part of the question is true. Because part of the statement is true and part is false, the question is misleading. A better question is:

(T F) A routine urinalysis specimen must be collected with clean technique.

True-false questions can be made more difficult by requiring the student to explain why the statement is true or false.

MATCHING QUESTIONS

Matching questions also test a low level of learning—that of knowledge. They are most useful for determining if students have learned definitions or equivalents of some type. They should be formatted in two columns, with the premise words or statements on the left and the definitions or responses on the right. You should have more responses than premises so that matching cannot be done simply by process of elimination. Instructions should be given that indicate whether responses can be used more than once or even not used at all. An example of a matching question is:

Match the definition on the right with the suffix on the left. Definitions can be used only once or not at all.

_____1.	_____-itis	a. presence of
_____2.	_____-stalsis	b. abnormal flow
_____3.	_____-rrhage	c. inflammation
_____4.	_____-iasis	d. discharge or flow
_____5.	_____-ectomy	e. contraction
		f. surgical removal of

MULTIPLE-CHOICE QUESTIONS

Multiple-choice questions can be written at the higher levels of knowing, from application through evaluation. At these higher levels they can test critical thinking. A multiple-choice question has two parts. The first part, the question, is also called the *stem*. The possible answers are called *options*. Among the options, the correct one is called the *answer*, while the incorrect options are termed *distracters*. You can word stems as questions or as incomplete statements that are completed by the options. For example, an item written as a question is:

WHAT IS A QUICK WAY TO ASSESS THE APPROXIMATE LITERACY LEVEL OF A PATIENT?

a. Pay attention to her vocabulary as she speaks.

b. Give her an instruction sheet to read.

c. Administer a literacy test.

d. Ask her whether she graduated from high school.

The same knowledge can be tested by a stem written as an incomplete statement:

A QUICK WAY TO ASSESS THE APPROXIMATE LITERACY LEVEL OF A PATIENT IS TO

a. pay attention to her vocabulary as she speaks.

b. give her an instruction sheet to read.

c. administer a literacy test.

d. ask her whether she graduated from high school.

Notice the differing formats used here. When the stem is a question, each option is capitalized. When the stem is an incomplete statement, it does not end with a period, so the options do not begin with a capital letter. This style may vary. In this manual's test bank, all options begin with a capital letter, regardless of whether the stem is a complete or incomplete sentence. Stems should be kept as brief as possible to minimize reading time. Avoid negatively stated stems. For example, a poor stem would be, "Which of the following is not a good way to assess a patient's literacy level?" It is too easy for readers to miss the word "not" and therefore answer incorrectly. If you feel compelled to write negative stems occasionally, be sure to capitalize or underline the word "not," or use the word "except," as in the following example: "All of the following are good ways to assess a patient's literacy level, EXCEPT." In this case, the reader is less likely to miss the negative word because of the sentence structure and also because the word "except" is capitalized.

Options usually vary from three to five in number. The more options you have, the more difficult the item. However, it is often difficult to write good distracters. Be sure that your options are grammatically consistent with the stem. Next is a test item in which all of the options do not fit grammatically with the stem:

THE LECTURE METHOD OF TEACHING IS BEST SUITED TO

a. when the audience already knows a lot about the topic.

b. large audiences.

c. times when you are in a hurry to cover your material and don't want to be interrupted.

d. young children.

Not only are the options grammatically inconsistent, they are also of varied lengths. Attempt to keep the options about the same length. The following restatement of the item corrects the problems with grammar and with length:

THE LECTURE METHOD OF TEACHING IS BEST SUITED TO

a. an audience that already knows the topic.

b. an audience that is very large.

c. times when you must cover your material quickly.

d. an audience of young children.

Distracters that make no sense should never be used. Instead, try to develop distracters that reflect incorrect ideas that some students might hold about a topic.

ESSAY QUESTIONS

Essay-type questions include short answer (restricted-response questions) and full essays (extended-response questions). These types of items can be used to test higher-order thinking. Extended-response essays are especially suited to testing analysis, synthesis, and evaluation levels of thinking. An example of an essay question that might test these higher-order levels of thinking is: "Explain how exogenous cortisone products mimic a person's normal cortisol functions and why long-term cortisone administration leads to complications. Also explain how nursing assessment and intervention can help to reduce those complications."

The educator must plan how the essay is going to be graded before the test is given. An outline of required facts and concepts can be developed and points given to each. Then a decision must be made as to whether it is appropriate to give points for writing style, grammar, spelling, and so on.

TEST ITEM ANALYSIS

After a test is given, an analysis of objective items can be conducted. Two common analyses are *item difficulty* and *item discrimination.* Most instructors want to develop questions that are of moderate difficulty, with around half of the students selecting the correct answer. A mixture of fairly easy, moderate, and difficult questions can be used.

The difficulty index can be easily calculated by dividing the number of students who answered the question correctly by the total number of students answering the question. The resulting fraction, converted to a percentage, gives an estimate of the difficulty, with lower percentages reflecting more difficult questions.

Item discrimination is an estimate of how well a particular item differentiates between students who generally know the material and those who don't. Another way of saying this is that a discriminating item is one that most of the students who got high scores on the rest of the examination got right and most of the students who got low scores got wrong. The discrimination index can be calculated by computer software or by hand using a formula that can be found in tests and measurement textbooks.

These few pages are but an introduction to teaching techniques. For more information, you might consult the following resources:

Book: DeYoung, S. (2003). *Teaching Strategies for Nurse Educators.* Upper Saddle River, NJ: Prentice Hall.

Websites:

www.crlt.umich.edu/tstrategies/teachings.html

www.gmu.edu/facstaff/part-time/strategy.html

www.ic.arizona.edu/ic/edtech/strategy.html

CHAPTER 1
CONTEMPORARY MATERNAL, NEWBORN, AND CHILD HEALTH NURSING

LEARNING OUTCOME 1

Identify the nursing roles available to maternal-newborn and pediatric nurses.

Concepts for Lecture

1. Registered nurses provide nursing care to both inpatient and outpatient women with childbearing or reproductive issues as well as newborns and children.
2. Nurse practitioners provide ambulatory care services to expectant families. They also function in some acute care and high-risk units.
3. Certified nurse-midwives manage the care of women who are at low risk for complications during pregnancy and childbirth.
4. Clinical nurse specialists (CNSs) have a master's degree and specialized knowledge and competence in a specific clinical area.

 POWERPOINT SLIDES 18–26

Figure 1–1. A certified nurse-midwife confers with her client

 SUGGESTION FOR CLASSROOM ACTIVITIES

- Assign students to work in groups. Allow each group to select one nursing specialty. Instruct members of the individual groups to review the educational preparation and responsibilities for each specialty. Allow each group to present the information to the class.

 SUGGESTION FOR CLINICAL ACTIVITIES

- Since client education is a major component of maternal child nursing, ask students to check the reading level of printed material used to educate children and families about a health condition. See if the printed material meets the fifth-grade reading equivalency.

LEARNING OUTCOME 2

Summarize the use of community-based nursing care in meeting the needs of childbearing and childrearing families.

Concepts for Lecture

1. Primary care includes a focus on health promotion, illness prevention, and individual responsibility for one's own health.
2. Community-based care is important in meeting the needs of the childbearing and childrearing family.
3. The vast majority of care takes place outside of the hospitals.

 POWERPOINT SLIDES 27–31

 SUGGESTION FOR CLASSROOM ACTIVITIES

- Instruct one group of students to list institutions where community-based services are performed. Instruct another group to list all the services that are available. Allow the students to match the cards according to institutions and services provided.

 SUGGESTION FOR CLINICAL ACTIVITIES

- Schedule students to obtain clinical experience in clinics, doctor's offices, and community organizations involved in providing maternal-child health care. Students may also be assigned to work with perinatal home health nurses.

LEARNING OUTCOME 3

Summarize the current status of factors related to health insurance and access to health care.

 POWERPOINT SLIDES 32–36

Concepts for Lecture

1. All pregnant women and children in the United States do not have access to health care.
2. Children living in poverty unable to receive basic preventive care.
3. Medicaid is most prevalent form of insurance among the poor.

LEARNING OUTCOME 4

Relate the availability of statistical data to the formulation of further research questions.

Concepts for Lecture

1. The birth rate in the United States increased for older women and decreased for teens.
2. Infant mortality rate is increasing in the United States.
3. Neonatal mortality rate increase is most prevalent during the first week of life.
4. Overall maternal mortality rate is decreasing in the United States.

LEARNING OUTCOME 5

Delineate significant legal and ethical issues that influence the practice of maternal-child nursing.

Concepts for Lecture

1. The fetus is increasingly viewed as a client separate from the mother. Human stem cells can be found in embryonic tissue and in the primordial germ cells of a fetus.
2. Abortion can legally be performed until the fetus reaches the age of viability. The decision to have an abortion is made by a woman in consultation with her physician.
3. Assisted reproductive technology (ART) is the term used to describe highly technologic approaches used to produce pregnancy.
4. Federal "Baby Doe" regulations were developed to protect the rights of infants with severe defects.

 SUGGESTION FOR CLASSROOM ACTIVITIES

- Allow students to discuss universal health care and the implications. Ask individuals in the classroom to say whether or not universal health care will increase access to health care for all. Allow them to provide evidence to support their conclusions.

 SUGGESTION FOR CLINICAL ACTIVITIES

- Have students research the requirement for Medicaid reimbursement and private insurance in a clinical facility. Allow them to compare and contrast the process.

 POWERPOINT SLIDES 37–42

Figure 1–3. Infant, neonatal, postneonatal mortality rates, United States, 1950–2005

 SUGGESTION FOR CLASSROOM ACTIVITIES

- Lead a discussion among students about the various factors that influence birth rates, neonatal mortality rates, infant mortality rates, and maternal mortality rates. For further review, advise students to visit the *mynursingkit.com* for cultural and statistical web links.

 SUGGESTION FOR CLINICAL ACTIVITIES

- Allow students to conduct research to identify the birth rate, neonatal mortality rate, infant mortality rate, and maternal mortality rate in their city or state according to race or ethnic origin. Discuss findings during postclinical conference.

 POWERPOINT SLIDES 43–49

 SUGGESTION FOR CLASSROOM ACTIVITIES

- Assign students to review the "Case Study: Cord Blood Banking" activity on *mynursingkit.com*

SUGGESTION FOR CLINICAL ACTIVITIES

- Assign students to an ethics committee meeting addressing quality of life issues in the perinatal environment. Students may also research past cases where federal regulations were considered and engage in active discussion during clinical conferences.

LEARNING OUTCOME 6

Discuss the role of evidence-based practice in improving the quality of nursing care for childbearing families.

Concepts for Lecture

1. Evidence-based practice refers to clinical practice based on research findings and other available data.
2. Evidence-based practice increases nurses' accountability and results in better client outcomes.

GENERAL CHAPTER CONSIDERATIONS

1. Have students study and learn key terms listed at beginning of chapter.
2. Have students complete end-of-chapter exercises either in their book or on the MyNursingKit website.
3. Use the Classroom Response Questions provided in PowerPoint to assess students prior to lecture.

 POWERPOINT SLIDES 50–53

 SUGGESTION FOR CLASSROOM ACTIVITIES

- Lead a discussion on the advantages of evidenced-based practice. Allow students to vocalize their views on that subject. For additional information, Web links, and activities, instruct students to visit *mynursingkit.com*

 SUGGESTION FOR CLINICAL ACTIVITIES

- Ask students to inquire about the utilization of evidenced-based practice in healthcare institutions during their clinical rotation. Allow them to discuss their findings with the other students in their clinical groups.

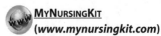 **MYNURSINGKIT**
(*www.mynursingkit.com*)

- NCLEX RN® review questions
- Case Studies
- Care Plans
- Critical Concept Review
- Thinking Critically
- Weblinks
- Weblink applications
- Nursing Tools
- Audio Glossary
- Images and Tables Library

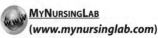 **MYNURSINGLAB**
(*www.mynursinglab.com*)

- Knowledge Quick Check
- Pre/Posttests
- Customized study plans
- Images and Tables Library
- *Separate purchase*

CLINICAL SKILLS MANUAL

- *Separate purchase*

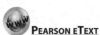 **PEARSON eTEXT**

- Students can search, highlight, take notes, and more all in electronic format
- *Separate purchase*

 TESTBANK

CHAPTER 2
CULTURE AND THE FAMILY

LEARNING OUTCOME 1

Distinguish among several different types of families.

Concepts for Lecture

1. A *family* is defined as individuals who are joined together by marriage, blood, adoption, or residence in the same household. More broadly, bonds of emotional closeness, sharing, and support generally characterize families.
2. There are numerous types of families that are both traditional and nontraditional.

LEARNING OUTCOME 2

Identify the stages of a family life cycle.

Concepts for Lecture

1. Duvall described an eight-stage family life cycle that describes the developmental process that each family encounters. It is based on the nuclear family, and the oldest child serves as the marker except in the last two stages when no children are present. Families with more than one child may overlap stages. Refer to Table 2-1 for details.
2. Other family models reflecting the contemporary family have been developed, but are outside the scope of this text.

 POWERPOINT SLIDES 21–32

Figure 2–1. Single-parent families account for nearly one third of all U.S. families

 SUGGESTIONS FOR CLASSROOM ACTIVITIES

- Pass around blank index cards and ask students to write the type of family they grew up in. Have them turn the cards in. Briefly tally the results of the group and share with the class.
- Review Figure 2-1. Ask students to compare and contrast the difficulties faced by single-parent and blended families.

 SUGGESTION FOR CLINICAL ACTIVITIES

- Remind students to explore the type of families their clients come from. This can make a tremendous difference in the nursing care provided, and families may not offer the information if they are not asked.

 POWERPOINT SLIDES 33–35

Table 2–1. Eight-stage family life cycle

 VIDEO CLIPS

Infant Massage

 SUGGESTION FOR CLASSROOM ACTIVITIES

- Divide the class into eight groups and assign each group one of the eight stages described in the lecture. Have each group identify the tasks and challenges faced by families during that stage. Have each group share their ideas with the class.

 SUGGESTION FOR CLINICAL ACTIVITIES

- Remind students to consider which stage the family they are caring for is in, as well as the tasks and challenges faced during this stage, and if the family has met these challenges.

LEARNING OUTCOME 3

Identify prevalent cultural norms related to childbearing and childrearing.

Concepts for Lecture

1. The culture that a family exists in has a great influence on childbearing practices, including the number of children a family has, the status conferred with the child's gender, and beliefs about contraception.
2. Cultures have different expectations of children, and these impact how families raise their children. *Refer to Table 2-3 for specific details.*

 POWERPOINT SLIDES 36–39

Table 2–3. Child rearing practices of selected cultures

 SUGGESTION FOR CLASSROOM ACTIVITIES

- Ask students to share cultural practices related to childbearing or childrearing that they have experienced in their own families.

 SUGGESTION FOR CLINICAL ACTIVITIES

- Discuss possible cultural beliefs that may conflict with nursing. For example, if a family wanted to light candles in their hospital room, how could the nurse address the situation? Why does the family believe that the ritual is important? Is there a way to compromise?

LEARNING OUTCOME 4

Summarize the importance of cultural competency in providing nursing care.

Concepts for Lecture

1. Cultural competency is the skills and knowledge necessary to appreciate, respect, and effectively work with individuals from different cultures. It requires self-awareness, an understanding of cultural differences, and the ability to adapt clinical practices into the family's belief system.
2. Biological differences include genetic and physical differences among cultural groups. These differences affect both nursing assessment and patterns of disease.
3. Communication is the method by which members of cultural groups share information. Although language is the most obvious form of communication, factors such as nonverbal communication, touch, and space are also important forms of communication.
4. Time orientation varies greatly among cultures. Cultural groups may place emphasis on events from the past, present, or future. The use of clocks may be limited in certain cultures.
5. Nutrition, and the role of food, plays a large part in many cultures. Nutritional assessments should take culture into account.

 POWERPOINT SLIDES 40–46

 SUGGESTION FOR CLASSROOM ACTIVITIES

- Ask students to discuss how culture impacts health literacy in maternal child nursing.

 SUGGESTION FOR CLINICAL ACTIVITIES

- Have students shadow a dietitian for part of a clinical day. Incorporate cultural preferences for food into the nutritional assessment.

LEARNING OUTCOME 5

Discuss the use of a cultural assessment tool as a means of providing culturally sensitive care.

Concepts for Lecture

1. Cultural assessment tools assist the nurse in gathering culturally appropriate information in a succinct, systematic way.

 POWERPOINT SLIDES 47–50

 SUGGESTION FOR CLASSROOM ACTIVITIES

- During class, have students read "Evidence-Based Nursing: Investigating Culture and Healthcare Barriers." Use the Critical Thinking questions at the end of the case to discuss how cultural assessment tools could be used to identify barriers to health care.

LEARNING OUTCOME 6

Identify key considerations in providing spiritually sensitive care.

Concepts for Lecture

1. *Religion* and *spirituality* mean different things to different people. The religious beliefs of families can influence their attitudes toward health care, childbearing, and childrearing.
2. There are several strategies that nurses can use to provide spiritually sensitive care. Self-awareness and respect are among the most important.

LEARNING OUTCOME 7

Distinguish between *complementary* and *alternative* therapies.

Concepts for Lecture

1. *Complementary therapies* are adjuncts to conventional medical treatments. They have been through scientific testing and have demonstrated some degree of reliability. Examples include acupuncture, acupressure, and massage therapy.
2. *Alternative therapies* are substances or procedures that are often used in place of conventional medical therapy. They may not have undergone rigorous scientific testing in the United States, but may have undergone testing in other countries.
3. Some examples of complementary and alternative therapies include homeopathy, naturopathy, traditional Chinese medicine, mind-based therapies, chiropractic, massage therapy, herbal therapy, and therapeutic touch.

LEARNING OUTCOME 8

Identify the benefits and risks of complementary and alternative therapies.

Concepts for Lecture

1. Complementary and alternative therapies have many potential benefits for women and children, including an emphasis on health promotion and wellness, low risk of side effects, and affordability.

SUGGESTION FOR CLINICAL ACTIVITIES

- Have students use the cultural assessment tools, which can be located on *mynursingkit.com* to assess a family they are caring for.

POWERPOINT SLIDES 51–56

SUGGESTION FOR CLASSROOM ACTIVITIES

- Have students identify religious beliefs of families that may conflict with the plan of care. Discuss strategies for accommodating these beliefs.

SUGGESTION FOR CLINICAL ACTIVITIES

- Members of Jehovah's Witness have hospital liaisons who work to educate healthcare providers about their belief system, as well as to use strategies that decrease the need for blood transfusion. If one of these liaisons exists in your community, invite them to attend clinical conference and discuss these topics with students. Although many students may not agree with the belief, they will have a better understanding of it.

POWERPOINT SLIDES 57–61

SUGGESTION FOR CLASSROOM ACTIVITIES

- Before class, divide students into groups and assign each group a complementary or alternative therapy discussed in the text. Have each group prepare a brief summary of the therapy, along with specific considerations regarding childbearing and childrearing families. Have each group present their findings to the class.

SUGGESTION FOR CLINICAL ACTIVITIES

- Some hospitals are becoming more accepting of complementary and alternative therapies. Determine what the policy is in your local clinical setting.

POWERPOINT SLIDES 62–65

SUGGESTION FOR CLASSROOM ACTIVITIES

- Identify specific herbs that should be avoided during pregnancy. Locate reliable resources on the Internet that students can use, and share these Web sites with the class.

2. Complementary and alternative therapies carry some risk to women and children, including lack of standardization, lack of research, and a poor understanding of potential side effects of some substances. Herbal therapy has particular risks for childbearing women.

LEARNING OUTCOME 9

Discuss complementary therapies appropriate for the nurse to use with childbearing and childrearing families.

Concepts for Lecture

1. Nurses who choose to use complementary and alternative therapies should only use methods that are within their scope of nursing practice. Therapies should generally be noninvasive and somewhat mainstream. Such therapies should be documented within the context of nursing practice.

GENERAL CHAPTER CONSIDERATIONS

1. Have students study and learn key terms listed at beginning of chapter.
2. Have students complete end-of-chapter exercises either in their book or on the MyNursingKit website.
3. Use the Classroom Response Questions provided in PowerPoint to assess students prior to lecture.

 SUGGESTION FOR CLINICAL ACTIVITIES

- As an alternative clinical experience, assign students to observe with a practitioner of alternative or complementary therapies. If students have never seen a chiropractic adjustment or an acupuncture session, it can be very revealing. They may be surprised to learn that many practitioners also treat women and children.

 POWERPOINT SLIDES 66–69

Figure 2–5. Infant massage

 SUGGESTION FOR CLASSROOM ACTIVITIES

- Assign groups of students to report on acupuncture, tai chi, and message therapy in maternal and child nursing. Review Figure 2-5 with the students.

 SUGGESTION FOR CLINICAL ACTIVITIES

- Determine if the hospital or clinical setting has a policy regarding nurses practicing complementary or alternative therapies.

 MYNURSINGKIT
(*www.mynursingkit.com*)

- NCLEX RN® review questions
- Case Studies
- Care Plans
- Critical Concept Review
- Thinking Critically
- Weblinks
- Weblink applications
- Nursing Tools
- Audio Glossary
- Images and Tables Library

 MYNURSINGLAB
(*www.mynursinglab.com*)

- Knowledge Quick Check
- Pre/Posttests
- Customized study plans
- Images and Tables Library
- *Separate purchase*

CLINICAL SKILLS MANUAL

- *Separate purchase*

 PEARSON eTEXT

- Students can search, highlight, take notes, and more all in electronic format
- *Separate purchase*

 TESTBANK

Chapter 3
Reproductive Anatomy and Physiology

Learning Outcome 1

Identify the structures and functions of the female reproductive system.

Concepts for Lecture

1. The female reproductive system consists of several organs that work together to facilitate ovulation, fertilization, implantation and fetal development, and birth.
2. Both male and female reproductive systems produce hormones and secretions to stimulate and support reproduction.

 PowerPoint Slides 20–27

Figure 3–2. Female external genitals, longitudinal view

Figure 3–3. Female internal reproductive organs

Activity: Female Reproductive System

 Suggestion for Classroom Activities

- Assign students to complete the activities: "Female Reproductive System" on *mynursingkit.com* and discuss in class.

 Suggestion for Clinical Activities

- Have students view the female pelvis animations on *mynursingkit.com*

Learning Outcome 2

Identify the structures and functions of the male reproductive system.

Concepts for Lecture

1. Male reproductive structures located in the pelvis and outside of the pelvis also play their part in reproduction.
2. Each structure works together to facilitate reproduction.
3. The male reproductive organs produce the germ cell and are responsible for transporting it to the site of reproduction.

 PowerPoint Slides 28–33

Figure 3–17. Male reproductive system, sagittal view

Figure 3–18. Schematic representation of a mature spermatozoon

 Animation

3-D Male Pelvis

Activity: Male Reproductive System

 Suggestion for Classroom Activities

- Instruct students to view animation of the male pelvis on the *mynursingkit.com*

 Suggestion for Clinical Activities

- Assign students to label a drawing of the male pelvis. Lead a discussion in the function of the male pelvis. Allow students to identify and discuss the functions of organs contained in the male pelvis.

LEARNING OUTCOME 3

Discuss the significance of specific female reproductive structures during childbirth.

Concepts for Lecture

1. The pelvic cavity is divided into the false pelvis and the true pelvis.
2. There are four basic pelvic types. Each type has a characteristic shape, and each shape has implications for labor and birth.

LEARNING OUTCOME 4

Summarize the actions of the hormones that affect reproductive functioning.

Concepts for Lecture

1. Estrogen stimulates and supports reproduction in a variety of ways and has several functions in the female reproductive system.
2. Progesterone causes increased proliferation and secretion of glandular tissue in the reproductive system. It is also responsible for decreasing myometrial contractility.
3. Prostaglandins also play a role in reproduction.

LEARNING OUTCOME 5

Identify the two phases of the ovarian cycle and the changes that occur in each phase.

 POWERPOINT SLIDES 34–38

Figure 3–9. Pelvic bones with supporting ligaments

 ANIMATION

3-D Female Pelvis

 SUGGESTION FOR CLASSROOM ACTIVITIES

- Allow students to review the female pelvis animation on *mynursingkit.com*

 SUGGESTION FOR CLINICAL ACTIVITIES

- Assign students to draw and label a diagram of the female pelvis. Allow students to identify the shape of a client's pelvis and discuss the impact on labor.

 POWERPOINT SLIDES 39–44

Figure 3–1. Physiologic changes leading to onset of puberty

Figure 3–14. Female reproductive cycle: interrelationships of hormones with the four phases of the uterine cycle and the two phases of the ovarian cycle in an ideal 28-day cycle

 SUGGESTION FOR CLASSROOM ACTIVITIES

- Allow students to use the *mynursingkit.com* to access the Reproductive Anatomy and Physiology Weblinks for further discussion and review, particularly on puberty. Review Figure 3-1 on puberty.

 SUGGESTION FOR CLINICAL ACTIVITIES

- Instruct students to go to *mynursingkit.com* and complete NCLEX questions. Have them visit the Reproductive Anatomy and Physiology Weblinks for further review before the next clinical day. Allow students to review NCLEX questions during pre- or postclinical conference.

 POWERPOINT SLIDES 45–50

Figure 3–14. Female reproductive cycle: interrelationships of hormones with the four phases of the uterine cycle and the two phases of the ovarian cycle in an ideal 28-day cycle

Concepts for Lecture

1. The ovarian cycle has two phases: the follicular phase (days 1 to 14) and the luteal phase (days 15 to 28 in a 28-day cycle). Figure 3-14 depicts the changes. Maturation of the ovarian follicle occurs in the follicular phase.
2. The corpus luteum develops during the luteal phase and secretes progesterone during the time the endometrium is favorable for implantation.

LEARNING OUTCOME 6

Describe the phases of the uterine (menstrual) cycle, their dominant hormones, and the changes that occur in each phase.

Concepts for Lecture

1. The menstrual phase is marked by hormonal changes and changes in the myometrium. Refer to Figure 3-14.
2. During the proliferative phase several changes take place in the endometrial glands, cervical mucus, and estrogen levels.
3. The secretory phase begins after ovulation and is influenced primarily by progesterone.
4. If fertilization does not occur, the ischemic phase begins. The corpus luteum begins to degenerate, and as a result both estrogen and progesterone levels fall.

Figure 3–15. Various stages of development of the ovarian follicles

Activity: Ovulation

SUGGESTION FOR CLASSROOM ACTIVITIES

- Assign students to participate in the Ovulation Activity on *mynursingkit.com* and discuss their findings.

SUGGESTION FOR CLINICAL ACTIVITIES

- Divide students into groups and assign each group to present to the rest of the class at least one aspect of ovulation. For example, one group may present the action of the FSH, another the LH hormone, and other groups may discuss the functions of individual hormones and the phases of the ovulation cycle.

POWERPOINT SLIDES 51–55

Figure 3–14. Female reproductive cycle: interrelationships of hormones with the four phases of the uterine cycle and the two phases of the ovarian cycle in an ideal 28-day cycle

SUGGESTION FOR CLASSROOM ACTIVITIES

- Engage students in critical thinking exercises on *mynursingkit.com*

SUGGESTION FOR CLINICAL ACTIVITIES

- Assign students to review "Critical Thinking in Action" on *mynursingkit.com*

GENERAL CHAPTER CONSIDERATIONS

1. Have students study and learn key terms listed at beginning of chapter.
2. Have students complete end of chapter exercises either in their book or on the MyNursingKit website.
3. Use the Classroom Response Questions provided in PowerPoint to assess students prior to lecture.

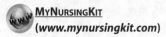

MyNursingKit
(*www.mynursingkit.com*)

- NCLEX RN® review questions
- Case Studies
- Care Plans
- Critical Concept Review
- Thinking Critically
- Weblinks
- Weblink applications
- Nursing Tools
- Audio Glossary
- Images and Tables Library

MyNursingLab
(*www.mynursinglab.com*)

- Knowledge Quick Check
- Pre/Posttests
- Customized study plans
- Images and Tables Library
- *Separate purchase*

CLINICAL SKILLS MANUAL

- *Separate purchase*

PEARSON eTEXT

- Students can search, highlight, take notes, and more all in electronic format
- *Separate purchase*

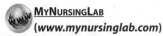

TESTBANK

CHAPTER 4
CONCEPTION AND FETAL DEVELOPMENT

LEARNING OUTCOME 1

Differentiate between meiotic cellular division and mitotic cellular division.

Concepts for Lecture

1. Each human begins life as a single cell called a fertilized ovum or zygote. Cells multiply through the process of cellular division. One type of cellular reproduction is called mitosis.
2. Meiosis is another process of cellular reproduction that is necessary for reproduction of the species.

 POWERPOINT SLIDES 24–31

Table 4–1. Comparison of meiosis and mitosis

 ANIMATION

Cell Division

 SUGGESTION FOR CLASSROOM ACTIVITIES

• Have students access *mynursingkit.com* to view the Cell Division animation and discuss in class.

 SUGGESTION FOR CLINICAL ACTIVITIES

• Allow students to draw labeled diagrams and discuss both types of cellular division. Refer to Table 4-1 when discussing.

LEARNING OUTCOME 2

Compare the processes by which ova and sperm are produced.

Concepts for Lecture

1. Oogenesis is a process that ends with the development of the ovum.
2. Spermatogenesis is the production of the male gamete or sperm. This process begins during puberty.

 POWERPOINT SLIDES 32–39

 ANIMATION

Oogenesis

 ANIMATION

Spermatogenesis

 ANIMATION

Oogenesis and Spermatogenesis Compared

Activity: Matching Oogenesis and Spermatogenesis

 SUGGESTION FOR CLASSROOM ACTIVITIES

• Instruct students to review the animations on Oogenesis, Spermatogenesis, Oogenesis and Spermatogenesis Compared, and Matching Oogenesis and Spermatogenesis, and discuss in class.

 SUGGESTION FOR CLINICAL ACTIVITIES

• Students may engage in a health teaching assignment related to the lecture topic in the clinical area.

LEARNING OUTCOME 3

Analyze the components of the process of fertilization as to how each may impact fertilization.

Concepts for Lecture

1. Preparation is the first component of fertilization.
2. Moment of fertilization is the second component of fertilization

 POWERPOINT SLIDES 40–47

Figure 4–2. Sperm penetration of an ovum. *A,* The sequential steps of oocyte penetration by a sperm are depicted moving from top to bottom. *B,* Scanning electron micrograph of a human sperm surrounding a human ovum (750X). The smaller spherical cells are granulosa cells of the corona radiata

Figure 4–3. Changes in fertilized ovum from conception to implantation. During ovulation the ovum leaves the ovary and enters the fallopian tube. Fertilization generally occurs in the outer third of the fallopian tube. Subsequent changes in the fertilized ovum from conception to implantation are depicted

 ANIMATION

Conception

 SUGGESTION FOR CLASSROOM ACTIVITIES

- Allow students to view conception animation on *mynursingkit.com*. To reinforce lecture information, assign from *mynursingkit.com* that students explore the Conception and Fetal Development Weblinks at home and attempt the critical thinking exercises.

 SUGGESTION FOR CLINICAL ACTIVITIES

- Have students review "Case Study: Teaching About Pregnancy" on *mynursingkit.com* and discuss the case study in pre- or post-clinical conference.

LEARNING OUTCOME 4

Analyze the processes that occur during the cellular multiplication and differentiation stages of intrauterine development and their effects on the structures that form.

Concepts for Lecture

1. Cellular multiplication begins as the zygote moves through the fallopian tube toward the cavity of the uterus.
2. About the 10th to 14th day after conception, the homogeneous mass of blastocyst cells differentiates into the primary germ layers. Refer to Table 4-3.

 POWERPOINT SLIDES 48–56

Table 4–2. Derivation of body structures from primary cell layers

Table 4–3. Timeline of organ system development in the embryo and fetus

Figure 4–4. Formation of primary germ layers

Figure 4–5. Differentiation of endoderm

 ANIMATION

Cell Division

 ANIMATION

Placenta Formation

LEARNING OUTCOME 5

Describe the development, structure, and functions of the placenta and umbilical cord during intrauterine life (embryonic and fetal development).

Concepts for Lecture

1. The umbilical cord connects the fetus to the placenta and facilitates fetal circulation.
2. The placenta allows metabolic and nutrient exchange between the embryonic and maternal circulations.

LEARNING OUTCOME 6

Compare the factors and processes by which fraternal (dizygotic) and identical (monozygotic) twins are formed.

Concepts for Lecture

1. Identical twins are unique in that they come from a single fertilized ovum.
2. Fraternal twins come from two separate fertilized ova. Dizygotic twinning increases with maternal age up to about age 35 and then decreases abruptly.

SUGGESTION FOR CLASSROOM ACTIVITIES

- Suggest that students review the Conception and Fetal Development Weblinks on *mynursingkit.com* and complete chapter NCLEX questions. Allow students to review the cell division animation on the *mynursingkit.com*

POWERPOINT SLIDES 57–64

Figure 4–8. Maternal side of placenta

Figure 4–9. Fetal side of placenta

ANIMATION

Placenta Formation

ANIMATION

Embryonic Heart Formation and Fetal Circulation

SUGGESTION FOR CLASSROOM ACTIVITIES

- Facilitate in-class review of the placenta formation and fetal circulation animations on *mynursingkit.com*

SUGGESTION FOR CLINICAL ACTIVITIES

- Assign students to identify the stage of development of the placenta and its current function when caring for prenatal clients. After observing a delivery, have students note which side of the placenta is the maternal and what side is the fetal side.

POWERPOINT SLIDES 65–73

Figure 4–7. *A*, Formation of fraternal twins. (Note separate placentas.) *B*, Formation of identical twins

SUGGESTION FOR CLASSROOM ACTIVITIES

- Use clay to demonstrate the different process between dizygotic and monozygotic twinning.

SUGGESTION FOR CLINICAL ACTIVITIES

- Assign "Care Plan Activity: Client Fearful of Multiple Gestation" found on *mynursingkit.com*

LEARNING OUTCOME 7

Summarize the significant changes in growth and development of the fetus in utero at 4, 6, 12, 16, 20, 24, 28, 36, and 40 weeks' gestation.

Concepts for Lecture

1. Significant changes take place in fetal development during weeks 4 through 16.
2. Progressive changes continue from 20 through 40 weeks.

POWERPOINT SLIDES 74–82

Figure 4–12. The embryo at 5 weeks

Figure 4–16. The fetus at 20 weeks weighs 435 to 465 g and measures about 19 cm

Table 4–4. Fetal development: what parents want to know

ANIMATION

Embryonic Heart Formation and Fetal Circulation

SUGGESTION FOR CLASSROOM ACTIVITIES

- Have students review the embryonic heart formation and circulation animation on the *mynursingkit.com* and discuss in class.

SUGGESTIONS FOR CLINICAL ACTIVITIES

- Instruct students to prepare a health teaching assignment about fetal development for clients during clinical rotation.
- During clinical, if experiencing prenatal clients, identify and document stage and system growth for the time period.

LEARNING OUTCOME 8

Identify the factors that influence congenital malformations of the various organ systems.

Concepts for Lecture

1. Factors may impact embryonic and fetal development. The growing organism is most vulnerable to hazardous agents during the pregnancy. See Table 4-5.

POWERPOINT SLIDES 83–84

Table 4–3. Timeline of organ system development in the embryo and fetus

Table 4–5. Developmental vulnerability timetable

SUGGESTION FOR CLASSROOM ACTIVITIES

- Ask the students to review the "Critical Thinking in Action" scenario and to complete the questions that follow. Lead a classroom discussion regarding the answers.

SUGGESTION FOR CLINICAL ACTIVITIES

- Assign the students to review Table 4-4 and Table 4-5. Discuss the nursing implications of the information contained in those tables in clinical conference. Compare and contrast essential information that the client needs to know.

GENERAL CHAPTER CONSIDERATIONS

1. Have students study and learn key terms listed at beginning of chapter.
2. Have students complete end-of-chapter exercises either in their book or on the MyNursingKit website.
3. Use the Classroom Response Questions provided in PowerPoint to assess students prior to lecture.

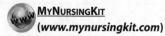

MyNursingKit
(www.mynursingkit.com)

- NCLEX RN® review questions
- Case Studies
- Care Plans
- Critical Concept Review
- Thinking Critically
- Weblinks
- Weblink applications
- Nursing Tools
- Audio Glossary
- Images and Tables Library

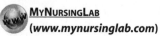

MyNursingLab
(www.mynursinglab.com)

- Knowledge Quick Check
- Pre/Posttests
- Customized study plans
- Images and Tables Library
- *Separate purchase*

CLINICAL SKILLS MANUAL

- *Separate purchase*

PEARSON eTEXT

- Students can search, highlight, take notes, and more all in electronic format
- *Separate purchase*

TESTBANK

CHAPTER 5
HEALTH PROMOTION FOR WOMEN

LEARNING OUTCOME 1

Determine accurate information to be provided to girls and women so that they can implement effective self-care measures for dealing with menstruation.

Concepts for Lecture

1. Nurses who work with young girls and adolescents can implement effective self-care measures for dealing with menstruation.
2. Nurses who work with teenagers need to provide basic information about menstruation.

LEARNING OUTCOME 2

Discriminate between the signs, symptoms, and nursing management of women with dysmenorrhea and premenstrual syndrome

Concepts for Lecture

1. Dysmenorrhea, or painful menstruation, occurs at, or a day before, the onset of menstruation and disappears by the end of menses.
2. Premenstrual syndrome (PMS) refers to a symptom complex associated with the luteal phase of the menstrual cycle (2 weeks prior to the onset of menses).

LEARNING OUTCOME 3

Compare the advantages, disadvantages, and effectiveness of the various methods of contraception available today.

Concepts for Lecture

1. There are various contraceptive methods with varying degrees of effectiveness. They can be described in terms of advantages, disadvantages, and effectiveness.

 POWERPOINT SLIDES 19–26

 SUGGESTION FOR CLINICAL ACTIVITIES

- Assign students to prepare a health teaching plan about menstruation to be used to teach adolescent clients in the clinical area.

 POWERPOINT SLIDES 27–34

 SUGGESTION FOR CLASSROOM ACTIVITIES

- Encourage students to explore additional interactive resources on *mynursingkit.com* through the Women's Health Weblinks in preparation for class lecture.

 SUGGESTION FOR CLINICAL ACTIVITIES

- Allow for clinical review of the Critical Thinking in Action case study in the textbook. Assign the students to develop patient teaching points for adolescents who have premenstrual syndrome.

 POWERPOINT SLIDES 35–50

Figure 5–1. The male condom. *A,* Unrolled condom with reservoir tip. *B,* Correct use of a condom

Figure 5–3. Inserting the diaphragm

Figure 5–4. Cervical cap

Figure 5–6. The Mirena Intrauterine System, which releases levonorgestrel gradually, may be left in place for up to 5 years

 ANIMATION
Oral Contraception

LEARNING OUTCOME 4

Delineate basic gynecologic screening procedures indicated for well women.

Concepts for Lecture

1. Monthly breast self-examination (BSE) is the best method for detecting breast masses.
2. A mammogram is a soft tissue x-ray of the breast that can detect lesions in the breast before they can be felt.
3. Pap smear detects cellular abnormalities at the cervix.
4. Pelvic examination allows for the detection of abnormalities of the reproductive organs and lower abdominal area. Refer to "Skill 2–2: Assisting with a Pelvic Exam" in the Skills Manual.

LEARNING OUTCOME 5

Consider the physical and psychologic aspects and clinical treatment options of menopause when caring for menopausal women.

Concepts for Lecture

1. During menopause the female experiences a variety of physical changes.
2. Psychological changes also affect the postmenopausal female.

SUGGESTION FOR CLASSROOM ACTIVITIES

• Assign students to review contraceptive agents on *mynursingkit.com*. Bring examples of various barrier methods of contraception to facilitate classroom discussion.

SUGGESTION FOR CLINICAL ACTIVITIES

• Assign students to a health clinic to shadow healthcare providers engaged in contraceptive counseling.

POWERPOINT SLIDES 51–66

Figure 5–8. Positions for inspection of the breasts

Figure 5–9. Procedure for breast self-examination

ANIMATION

Introduction to Mammography

SUGGESTION FOR CLASSROOM ACTIVITIES

• Discuss thin prep cytology method and its advantages.

SUGGESTION FOR CLINICAL ACTIVITIES

• Assign students to women's health clinics. Allow them to observe healthcare providers performing and assisting with pelvic examinations.

POWERPOINT SLIDES 67–75

SUGGESTION FOR CLASSROOM ACTIVITIES

• Assign students to review sexual needs of a menopausal women and nursing implications.
• In class, develop a teaching plan for a woman who is sexually active during menopause.

SUGGESTION FOR CLINICAL ACTIVITIES

• Suggest that students review "Complementary Care: Use of Botanicals for Menopausal Symptoms." Encourage them to access the Women's Health Weblinks for additional information. Allow students to observe postmenopausal counseling at a women's health clinic or doctor's office.

LEARNING OUTCOME 6

Delineate the nurse's role in screening and caring for women who have experienced domestic violence or rape.

Concepts for Lecture

1. The nurse caring for a victim of violence or rape functions in a variety of roles.
2. Battering takes place in a cyclic fashion through three phases.
3. Early identification of battered females and treatment is indicated for all females facing physical violence and psychological abuse. See Figure 5-10.

GENERAL CHAPTER CONSIDERATIONS

1. Have students study and learn key terms listed at beginning of chapter.
2. Have students complete end-of-chapter exercises either in their book or on the MyNursingKit website.
3. Use the Classroom Response Questions provided in PowerPoint to assess students prior to lecture.

 POWERPOINT SLIDES 76–79

Figure 5–10. Domestic violence screening

 VIDEO CLIPS

Spousal Abuse

 SUGGESTIONS FOR CLASSROOM ACTIVITIES

- Identify a specially trained sexual assault nurse examiner (SANE) in your community. Invite her to talk about her role in the community in relation to the care of victims of violence or rape in your classroom.
- Have students view the video on spousal abuse on *mynursingkit.com*. Utilize role play in the classroom to assist students in identifying the behavior of the abuser and the victim.

 SUGGESTIONS FOR CLINICAL ACTIVITIES

- Identify case studies of female victims of violence or rape. Allow students to participate in open discussion. Let them explore strategies to decrease domestic violence and rape.
- Schedule students to visit a homeless shelter for abused and battered women. Allow them to observe the activities that the clients engage in and the counseling that they receive.

 MYNURSINGKIT
(www.mynursingkit.com)

- NCLEX RN® review questions
- Case Studies
- Care Plans
- Critical Concept Review
- Thinking Critically
- Weblinks
- Weblink applications
- Nursing Tools
- Audio Glossary
- Images and Tables Library

 MYNURSINGLAB
(www.mynursinglab.com)

- Knowledge Quick Check
- Pre/Posttests
- Customized study plans
- Images and Tables Library
- *Separate purchase*

CLINICAL SKILLS MANUAL

- *Separate purchase*

 PEARSON ETEXT

- Students can search, highlight, take notes, and more all in electronic format
- *Separate purchase*

 TESTBANK

CHAPTER 6
COMMON GYNECOLOGIC PROBLEMS

LEARNING OUTCOME 1

Contrast the contributing factors, signs and symptoms, treatment options, and nursing care management of women with common benign breast disorders.

Concepts for Lecture

1. Fibrocystic breast changes, the most common of the benign breast disorders, are most prevalent in women 30 to 50 years of age.
2. Fibroadenoma is a common benign tumor seen in women in their teens and early 20s. It is potentially malignant.
3. Intraductal papillomas are tumors in the terminal portion of a duct associated with menopause.
4. Duct ectasis (comedomastitis) is an inflammatory condition of the ducts behind the nipple commonly occurring during or near the onset of menopause.

 POWERPOINT SLIDES 25–32

 SUGGESTION FOR CLASSROOM ACTIVITIES

- In class have students engage in role play and vocalize specific signs and symptoms of each benign breast disorder. Students may be assigned to play the role of the clients with the various conditions or the healthcare provider recommending treatment options.

 SUGGESTIONS FOR CLINICAL ACTIVITIES

- Arrange for students to spend several hours in a breast health clinic. Encourage students to observe the different screening procedures as well as the emotional reactions of the clients.
- Contact a school nurse who works with high school students. Arrange for nursing students to present a class on breast self-examination techniques to either female junior or senior high school students. The class would include a discussion on the importance of breast self-exam and a demonstration/practice session using a breast self-exam model.

LEARNING OUTCOME 2

Consider the signs and symptoms, medical therapy, and implications for fertility in determining the nursing care management of women with endometriosis.

Concepts for Lecture

1. Endometriosis is a condition characterized by the presence of endometrial tissue outside of the uterine cavity. It may occur at any age after puberty, but is most common in women between ages 20 and 45. The most common symptom is pelvic pain.
2. Treatment may be medical, surgical, or a combination of the two.
3. The condition is often diagnosed when the woman seeks evaluation for infertility.

 POWERPOINT SLIDES 33–40

 SUGGESTION FOR CLASSROOM ACTIVITIES

- Discuss pharmacologic treatment of endometriosis and the nursing implications.

 SUGGESTION FOR CLINICAL ACTIVITIES

- Arrange for students to attend a self-help group for women who experience endometriosis.

LEARNING OUTCOME 3

Identify the risk factors, treatment options, and nursing interventions for a woman with toxic shock syndrome.

Concepts for Lecture

1. Toxic shock syndrome (TSS) is primarily a disease of women at or near menses or during the postpartum period. The causative organism is *Staphylococcus aureus*. Several factors place the woman at risk for this condition.
2. Early diagnosis and treatment are important in preventing death.
3. Education of women is key to preventing toxic shock syndrome (TSS).

LEARNING OUTCOME 4

Compare the causes, signs and symptoms, treatment options, and nursing care for women with vulvovaginal candidiasis versus bacterial vaginosis.

Concepts for Lecture

1. Signs and symptoms of vaginitis are the most common reasons women seek gynecologic care.
2. It may be caused by an infection or by an alteration of normal flora, as in the case of bacterial vaginosis and *Candida albicans*. Refer also to Drug Guide: Metronidazole, in *Maternal & Child Nursing Care*, 3/e.

LEARNING OUTCOME 5

Compare the prevention, causes, treatment options, and nursing care of women for the common sexually transmitted infections.

Concepts for Lecture

1. Sexually transmitted infections (STIs) are the most common reasons for outpatient, community-based treatment of women. Trichomoniasis is an infection caused by a microscopic motile protozoan.
2. Chlamydial infection is the most common bacterial STI in the United States. Gonorrhea is an infection also of bacterial origin.

 POWERPOINT SLIDES 41–46

 SUGGESTIONS FOR CLASSROOM ACTIVITIES

- Recommend that students review *mynursingkit.com* for resources related to toxic shock syndrome. Encourage students to access the Planned Parenthood website for information related to toxic shock syndrome and contraceptive agents.
- Divide the students into two groups. Have one group go online to find statistics regarding the incidence and mortality rate associated with toxic shock syndrome in the United States. Have another group go online to obtain information from two tampon manufacturers regarding the self-care measures that women can utilize to prevent TSS. In class, each group will present their findings.

 POWERPOINT SLIDES 47–58

Figure 6–1. Clue cells characteristically seen in bacterial vaginosis

Figure 6–2. The hyphae and spores of *Candida albicans*

 SUGGESTIONS FOR CLASSROOM ACTIVITIES

- For homework have students complete the NCLEX-RN® review questions. Review Metronidazole (Flagyl).
- Ask students to develop key patient teaching points related to metronidazole.

 SUGGESTION FOR CLINICAL ACTIVITIES

- Assign students to clinical areas where females commonly seek health care for vaginal infections. Allow students to teach clients how to prevent vaginal infections.

 POWERPOINT SLIDES 59–83

Figure 6–3. Microscopic appearance of *Trichomonas vaginalis*

Figure 6–4. Condylomata acuminata on the vulva

 VIDEO CLIPS

Acyclovir

3. Herpes genitalia is caused by a virus. Condylomata acuminata (venereal warts) is relatively common. This infection is also caused by a virus. Another sexually transmitted infection of viral origin is acquired immunodeficiency syndrome (AIDS).
4. Syphilis is a chronic STI caused by a spirochete.

SUGGESTIONS FOR CLASSROOM ACTIVITIES

- Invite a nurse from the county/state STI clinic to come to class to speak about strategies for working with clients with an STI.
- Encourage students to review "Teaching Highlights: Preventing STIs and Their Consequences" before the lecture. Allow open class discussion following the lecture.

SUGGESTIONS FOR CLINICAL ACTIVITIES

- If possible, assign at least one or two students to clients with STI. Allow them to discuss the nursing management of the individual clients during postclinical conference.
- Assign students into groups. Instruct each group to select a sexually transmitted disease and to formulate a teaching plan and present it to a group of clients.

LEARNING OUTCOME 6

Relate the implications of pelvic inflammatory disease (PID) for future fertility to its pathology, signs and symptoms, treatment, and nursing care.

Concepts for Lecture

1. The greatest problem of pelvic inflammatory disease is postinfection tubal damage often caused by chlamydia and gonorrhea.
2. The woman who is acutely ill will have obvious signs and symptoms. A low-grade infection may be more difficult to detect.
3. Several combinations of therapy are utilized to treat this condition.
4. Women of reproductive age are most at risk for pelvic inflammatory disease.

POWERPOINT SLIDES 84–91

SUGGESTION FOR CLASSROOM ACTIVITIES

- Divide students into two groups. Have one group go online to determine what the PID occurrence rate is for each state and county in which the school is located. Have the second group go online to see what alternative/complementary treatment measures are available for PID treatment. Plan class time to discuss their findings.

SUGGESTION FOR CLINICAL ACTIVITIES

- If possible, assign one or two students to care for clients diagnosed with pelvic inflammatory disease. Allow students caring for the clients to present information about the medical and nursing management of the clients. Instruct them to compare this information with the information obtained in the lecture and the book.

LEARNING OUTCOME 7

Identify the cause and implications of an abnormal finding during a pelvic examination in the provision of nursing care.

Concepts for Lecture

1. A Papanicolaou (Pap) smear is a test done to screen for the presence of cellular anomalies of the cervix and cervical cancer.
2. Ovarian masses may be palpated during the pelvic examinations.
3. Fibroid tumors/leiomyomas are the most common benign uterine mass in women.
4. Endometrial cancer, most commonly a disease of postmenopausal women, has a high rate of cure if detected early.

POWERPOINT SLIDES 92–105

Table 6–1. The Bethesda System for classifying pap smears

SUGGESTIONS FOR CLASSROOM ACTIVITIES

- Have students refer to Table 6-1: The Bethesda System for Classifying Pap Smears, which is available on the *mynursingkit.com*
- Invite students to share experiences of their first pelvic exam in class. Allow students to discuss methods that could be used to decrease a client's anxiety regarding her first pelvic exam.

LEARNING OUTCOME 8

Contrast the causes, signs and symptoms, treatment options, and nursing care for women with cystitis versus pyelonephritis.

Concepts for Lecture

1. Cystitis is an infection of the lower urinary tract or the bladder.
2. Pyelonephritis is an infection of the upper urinary tract or the kidneys.

GENERAL CHAPTER CONSIDERATIONS

1. Have students study and learn key terms listed at beginning of chapter.
2. Have students complete end-of-chapter exercises either in their book or on the MyNursingKit website.
3. Use the Classroom Response Questions provided in PowerPoint to assess students prior to lecture.

 SUGGESTIONS FOR CLINICAL ACTIVITIES

- Provide pelvic models and speculums for student practice.
- Discuss the implications of HPV and an abnormal pap smear.

 POWERPOINT SLIDES 106–111

 SUGGESTIONS FOR CLASSROOM ACTIVITIES

- In-class review of "Teaching Highlights: Preventing Cystitis."
- Divide students into pairs and let them practice teaching each other ways to avoid cystitis.

 SUGGESTION FOR CLINICAL ACTIVITIES

Allow students to utilize "Teaching Highlights: Preventing Cystitis" in the clinical area as a health teaching tool for clients at the clinical site.

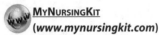 **MYNURSINGKIT** (*www.mynursingkit.com*)

- NCLEX RN® review questions
- Case Studies
- Care Plans
- Critical Concept Review
- Thinking Critically
- Weblinks
- Weblink applications
- Nursing Tools
- Audio Glossary
- Images and Tables Library

 MYNURSINGLAB (*www.mynursinglab.com*)

- Knowledge Quick Check
- Pre/Posttests
- Customized study plans
- Images and Tables Library
- *Separate purchase*

CLINICAL SKILLS MANUAL

- *Separate purchase*

 PEARSON ETEXT

- Students can search, highlight, take notes, and more all in electronic format
- *Separate purchase*

 TESTBANK

CHAPTER 7
FAMILIES WITH SPECIAL REPRODUCTIVE CONCERNS

LEARNING OUTCOME 1

Identify the essential components of fertility.

Concepts for Lecture

1. Essential components present in the female are vital for fertility.
2. There are elements in the male that facilitate fertility.

POWERPOINT SLIDES 20–26

Table 7–1. Possible causes of infertility

Table 7–2. Initial infertility physical workup and laboratory evaluations

VIDEO CLIPS

What Is a Gene?

Activity: Ovulation

SUGGESTIONS FOR CLASSROOM ACTIVITIES

• Facilitate an in-class review of "Complementary Care: Common Treatments for Infertility" and Tables 7–1 and 7–2.
• Have students do the Ovulation activity on *mynursingkit.com*

SUGGESTION FOR CLINICAL ACTIVITIES

• Assign the "Critical Thinking in Action" to review on *mynursingkit.com* and completion of questions on Fertility Awareness.

LEARNING OUTCOME 2

Describe the elements of the preliminary investigation of infertility and the nurse's role in supporting/teaching clients during this phase.

Concepts for Lecture

1. There are several elements to consider when performing a preliminary investigation of the infertile couple. Refer to Table 7–3.
2. A fertility problem is a deeply personal, emotion-laden area in a couple's life.

POWERPOINT SLIDES 27–32

Figure 7–1. Flow chart for management of the infertile couple

Table 7–3. Normal semen analysis

SUGGESTIONS FOR CLASSROOM ACTIVITIES

• Recommend students prepare for an in-class discussion about "Case Study: Infertility" by reviewing the activity on *mynursingkit.com*
• Invite a nurse practitioner who works with infertile couples to speak on the elements of the initial infertility assessment.

SUGGESTION FOR CLINICAL ACTIVITIES

• Assign students the care plan activity on *mynursingkit.com*, "Infertile Couple," in preparation for clinical discussion.

Learning Outcome 3

Summarize the indications for the tests and associated treatments, including assisted reproductive technologies, that are done in an infertility workup.

Concepts for Lecture

1. There are several indications for tests and treatments for infertility.

Learning Outcome 4

Relate the physiologic and psychologic effects of infertility on a couple to the nursing management of the couple.

Concepts for Lecture

1. Infertility therapy taxes a couple's financial, physical, and psychological resources.

Learning Outcome 5

Describe the nurse's role as counselor, educator, and advocate for couples during infertility evaluation and treatment.

Concepts for Lecture

1. As nurses care for infertile couples, they function in a variety of roles.

 PowerPoint Slides 33–41

Table 7–4. Drugs commonly used to treat infertility

 Suggestions for Classroom Activities

- Utilize the infertility questionnaire as a tool for students to use during a role play depicting an infertile couple at their first interview.
- Divide students into groups of three or four. Assign each group a different pharmacological agent used to manage infertility. Have each group present information related to the purpose, mechanism of action, side effects, and nursing considerations. Allow time for students to present their findings.

 Suggestion for Clinical Activities

- Discuss priority teaching when a client is on Danocrine and/or ovulation-induction agents.

 PowerPoint Slides 42–45

 Suggestions for Classroom Activities

- Assign the chapter NCLEX review questions for students to complete prior to class.
- Divide the class in three groups and have each group develop three priority nursing diagnoses and expected outcomes for a client experiencing infertility.

 Suggestion for Clinical Activities

- Students may access the Reproductive Weblinks on *mynursingkit.com* for additional information in preparation for postclinical conference.

 PowerPoint Slides 46–49

 Suggestion for Classroom Activities

- Invite a registered nurse or nurse practitioner who specializes in caring for infertile couples to speak to your class about the roles of nurses caring for infertile couples.

 Suggestion for Clinical Activities

- Arrange for students to rotate to a fertility clinic. Assign them to observe the various roles that nurses play in the management of infertility. Allow them to discuss their observations during post-clinical conference.

LEARNING OUTCOME 6

Identify couples who may benefit from preconceptual chromosomal analysis and prenatal testing when providing care to couples with special reproductive concerns.

Concepts for Lecture

1. Preconceptual chromosomal analysis and prenatal testing is important to identify congenital abnormalities and chromosomal defects.

POWERPOINT SLIDES 50–56

SUGGESTIONS FOR CLASSROOM ACTIVITIES

- Assign students to gather additional information about genetic testing like the Human Genome Project from Weblinks at *mynursingkit.com*. Allow class discussion of information gathered.
- Invite a couple or a parent who have a child with a genetic defect to share their experience with the class. Prior to class, have students learn about the genetic defect that the couple or a parent will be discussing.

SUGGESTION FOR CLINICAL ACTIVITIES

- Arrange for students to rotate to a clinic that screens for birth defects and provides counseling and treatment options for clients. Allow them to observe the process from admission through testing and counseling.

LEARNING OUTCOME 7

Identify the characteristics of autosomal dominant, autosomal recessive, and X-linked (sex-linked) recessive disorders.

Concepts for Lecture

1. A person is said to have an autosomal dominantly inherited disorder if the disease trait is heterozygous; that is, the abnormal gene overshadows the normal gene of the pair to produce the trait.
2. In an autosomal recessive inherited disorder, the person must have two abnormal genes to be affected.
3. X-linked, or sex-linked, disorders are those for which the abnormal gene is carried on the X chromosome. Refer to Figure 7-16.

POWERPOINT SLIDES 57–66

Figure 7–14. Autosomal dominant pedigree

Figure 7–15. Autosomal recessive pedigree

Figure 7–16. X-linked recessive pedigree

SUGGESTION FOR CLASSROOM ACTIVITIES

- Invite a healthcare provider who specializes in genetic disorders to talk to students about the prevalence and management of genetic disorders.

SUGGESTION FOR CLINICAL ACTIVITIES

- Arrange for clinical rotation at a genetic clinic. In preparation for clinical conference, advise students to complete the NCLEX-RN® review questions and to review the Web links for this chapter on *mynursingkit.com*

LEARNING OUTCOME 8

Compare prenatal and postnatal diagnostic procedures used to determine the presence of genetic disorders.

Concepts for Lecture

1. The ability to diagnose certain genetic diseases has enormous implications for the practice of preventive health care. Several methods are available for prenatal diagnosis. Refer to "Skill 2-5: Assisting During Amniocentesis" in the Clinical Skills Manual.

POWERPOINT SLIDES 67–74

Figure 7–17 (A&B). *A,* Genetic amniocentesis. This method used for prenatal diagnosis is done at 14 to 16 weeks' gestation. *B,* Chorionic villus sampling is done at 8 to 10 weeks, and the cells are karyotyped within 48 to 72 hours

Figure 7–18 (A&B). Dermatoglyphic patterns of the hands

2. When a child is born with anomalies, has a stormy newborn period, or does not progress as expected, a genetic evaluation may be warranted during the postnatal period.

LEARNING OUTCOME 9

Explore the emotional impact on a couple undergoing genetic testing or coping with the birth of a baby with a genetic disorder and explain the nurse's role in supporting the family undergoing genetic counseling.

Concepts for Lecture

1. Parents experience grief, fear, and anger when they discover that their baby has been born with a defect or a genetic disease.
2. The nurse's role involves clarifying issues for the family.

SUGGESTION FOR CLASSROOM ACTIVITIES

• When preparing for lecture, advise students to review "Skill 2-5: Assisting During Amniocentesis," in the Clinical Skills Manual. Review with students priority nursing intervention before the procedure and after the procedure.

SUGGESTION FOR CLINICAL ACTIVITIES

• Assign students to prenatal testing centers. Facilitate their involvement in caring for clients having genetic tests. Arrange to have students discuss their observations and experiences during postclinical conference.

POWERPOINT SLIDES 75–78

SUGGESTION FOR CLASSROOM ACTIVITIES

• Invite a registered nurse or nurse practitioner who is experienced in caring for clients who require genetic testing to talk to your students about the emotional impact to clients and the roles nurses play when caring for those clients.

SUGGESTION FOR CLINICAL ACTIVITIES

• Arrange for students to shadow a healthcare provider at a genetic clinic. Allow them to follow clients through the initial assessment and follow-up. Discuss the indication of First Trimester Screen in clinical conference.

GENERAL CHAPTER CONSIDERATIONS

1. Have students study and learn key terms listed at beginning of chapter.
2. Have students complete end-of-chapter exercises either in their book or on the MyNursingKit website.
3. Use the Classroom Response Questions provided in PowerPoint to assess students prior to lecture.

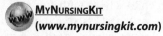 **MYNURSINGKIT**
(*www.mynursingkit.com*)

- NCLEX RN® review questions
- Case Studies
- Care Plans
- Critical Concept Review
- Thinking Critically
- Weblinks
- Weblink applications
- Nursing Tools
- Audio Glossary
- Images and Tables Library

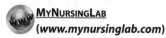 **MYNURSINGLAB**
(*www.mynursinglab.com*)

- Knowledge Quick Check
- Pre/Posttests
- Customized study plans
- Images and Tables Library
- *Separate purchase*

CLINICAL SKILLS MANUAL

- *Separate purchase*

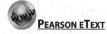 **PEARSON eTEXT**

- Students can search, highlight, take notes, and more all in electronic format
- *Separate purchase*

 TESTBANK

Chapter 8
Preparation for Parenthood

Learning Outcome 1

Determine the most appropriate nursing care for couples during preconception to help ensure their best possible health state.

Concepts for Lecture

1. Information is a major nursing responsibility during preconception counseling. Preconception counseling is necessary to assist couples in taking steps to ensure that they are in the best possible physical and mental health when pregnancy occurs.

PowerPoint Slides 20–25

Suggestion for Classroom Activities

- Assign students to search the Internet or a health data base for the Ayurvedic Diet and how it may relate to preconception care, and "Complementary Care: Ayurveda and Preconception Lifestyle" in the text. Facilitate an in-class discussion of ayurveda and preconception care.

Suggestion for Clinical Activities

- Arrange for students to attend a preconception class. Prior to this rotation, assign students to review lifestyle hazards and fertility concerns that impact conception.

Learning Outcome 2

Identify ways to assist expectant parents in making the best decisions possible about issues related to pregnancy, labor, and birth.

Concepts for Lecture

1. Couples are faced with making decisions about a multitude of issues related to pregnancy and the birthing process. Refer to Table 8-1.

PowerPoint Slides 26–30

Table 8–1. Benefits and risks of some consumer decisions during pregnancy, labor, and birth

Suggestions for Classroom Activities

- Provide examples of birthing plans for students to view.
- Invite a certified nurse-midwife who works at a birthing center to talk to the class about her or his role. Ask the midwife to discuss the advantages and differences between delivering a newborn at a birthing center or at an acute care setting.

Suggestion for Clinical Activities

- Have students review birthing plan calculators on the Internet and compare and contrast them to the information in Table 8-1.

Learning Outcome 3

Summarize the goals and content of the various types of antepartal education programs when providing nursing care for expectant couples and their families.

PowerPoint Slides 31–37

Figure 8–2. In a group setting with a nurse-instructor, expectant parents share information about pregnancy and childbirth

Concepts for Lecture

1. Prenatal education programs provide important opportunities to share information about pregnancy and childbirth and to enhance the parents' decision-making skills.
2. Prenatal classes are often divided into early and late classes.

LEARNING OUTCOME 4

Compare methods of childbirth preparation and the nursing interventions for each.

Concepts for Lecture

1. There are many different methods to prepare clients for childbirth. They all emphasize measures that help to decrease anxiety and pain. Refer to Table 8-3.
2. The nurse needs to be familiar with commonly used childbirth preparation methods and prepared to support the approach family has chosen.

 SUGGESTIONS FOR CLASSROOM ACTIVITIES

- Select students from the class to present and facilitate class discussion of information available on the March of Dimes website for childbearing families.
- Invite a lactation consultant to class to share her experiences providing breastfeeding teaching sessions to expectant couples. Ask the speaker to include information regarding the cost of classes, class content, and class length/duration.

 SUGGESTION FOR CLINICAL ACTIVITIES

- Arrange for students to attend a childbirth education class: sibling preparation, adolescent, childbirth preparation.

 POWERPOINT SLIDES 38–43

Figure 8–4. Effleurage is light stroking of the abdomen with the fingertips

Table 8–3. Summary of Selected Childbirth Preparation Methods

 VIDEO CLIPS

Effleurage Massage

 SUGGESTIONS FOR CLASSROOM ACTIVITIES

- Allow in-class review of Table 8-3. Ask students to identify the differences and the similarities of each method.
- Have students bring pillows and blankets to class. Divide students into groups of two—one student will be the coach, the other student the pregnant woman. Acting as the childbirth educator, have students practice progressive relaxation exercises, touch relaxation, effleurage, and two breathing techniques.
- Have students view the video Effleurage Massage.

 SUGGESTION FOR CLINICAL ACTIVITIES

- Assign students to labor and delivery. Select one group of students to care for clients who had no childbirth preparation classes. Assign another group to clients who had childbirth preparation classes. During postclinical conference allow students to describe, compare, and contrast clients' coping behavior during the birthing process.

LEARNING OUTCOME 5

Explore ways in which the nurse conveys respect for client individuality in preparing for childbirth.

Concepts for Lecture

1. Nurses must convey respect for clients during childbirth preparation classes.

GENERAL CHAPTER CONSIDERATIONS

1. Have students study and learn key terms listed at beginning of chapter.
2. Have students complete end-of-chapter exercises either in their book or on the MyNursingKit website.
3. Use the Classroom Response Questions provided in PowerPoint to assess students prior to lecture.

 POWERPOINT SLIDES 44–47

 SUGGESTIONS FOR CLASSROOM ACTIVITIES

- Suggest that students review "Developing Cultural Competence: Birth Choices" from the text in preparation for in-class discussion. Allow students to explain how cultural competence can assist in conveying respect to clients when teaching childbirth preparation classes.
- Invite a massage therapist, reflexologist, acupuncturist, and hypnotist to speak to the class on how their techniques provide comfort and pain reduction to the laboring woman. Ask the speakers to demonstrate their technique(s) in class.

 SUGGESTION FOR CLINICAL ACTIVITIES

- Assign a group of students to a prenatal clinic. Instruct students to prepare a childbirth preparation teaching plan for presentation at the clinic.

 MYNURSINGKIT
(www.mynursingkit.com)

- NCLEX RN® review questions
- Case Studies
- Care Plans
- Critical Concept Review
- Thinking Critically
- Weblinks
- Weblink applications
- Nursing Tools
- Audio Glossary
- Images and Tables Library

 MYNURSINGLAB
(www.mynursinglab.com)

- Knowledge Quick Check
- Pre/Posttests
- Customized study plans
- Images and Tables Library
- *Separate purchase*

CLINICAL SKILLS MANUAL

- *Separate purchase*

 PEARSON ETEXT

- Students can search, highlight, take notes, and more all in electronic format
- *Separate purchase*

 TESTBANK

CHAPTER 9
PHYSICAL AND PSYCHOLOGIC CHANGES OF PREGNANCY

LEARNING OUTCOME 1

Identify the anatomic and physiologic changes that occur during pregnancy.

Concepts for Lecture

1. Several anatomic and physiologic changes take place during pregnancy.

 POWERPOINT SLIDES 21–31

 SUGGESTION FOR CLASSROOM ACTIVITIES

- Provide a drawing of the female anatomy showing all organ systems. Instruct students to highlight each organ system that is affected during pregnancy, label each organ, and list the changes that occur in each organ system.

 SUGGESTION FOR CLINICAL ACTIVITIES

- Have students attend prenatal appointments with several women. In postconference, identify different system alterations in the three trimesters.

LEARNING OUTCOME 2

Assess the subjective (presumptive), objective (probable), and diagnostic (positive) changes of pregnancy in clients.

Concepts for Lecture

1. Many of the changes women experience during pregnancy are used to diagnose the pregnancy itself. They are called the subjective, or presumptive, changes; the objective, or probable, changes; and the diagnostic, or positive, changes of pregnancy. Refer to the "Nursing Practice" boxes in Chapter 9 of *Maternal & Child Nursing Care, 3rd ed.*

 POWERPOINT SLIDES 32–38

Figure 9–4. Hegar's sign

Table 9–1. Differential diagnosis of pregnancy—subjective changes

Table 9–2. Differential diagnosis of pregnancy—objective changes

 SUGGESTION FOR CLASSROOM ACTIVITIES

- Ask for a volunteer who has been pregnant from your group of students to share her experience with the rest of the class. Allow her to highlight the subjective and presumptive signs and symptoms that she experienced. Allow students to use Tables 9-1 and 9-2 to develop a list of differential diagnoses relative to the information that the selected student provides.

 SUGGESTIONS FOR CLINICAL ACTIVITIES

- Schedule students to rotate to an antepartum unit or prenatal clinic. Select a client and demonstrate the positive signs of pregnancy. Allow students to listen to the fetal heart rate, palpate fetal movements, and visualize the fetus via ultrasound.
- Assign students to complete "Critical Thinking in Action" at the end of Chapter 9. Discuss answers in clinical conference.

LEARNING OUTCOME 3

Contrast the various types of pregnancy tests.

Concepts for Lecture

1. A variety of assay techniques are available to detect hCG during early pregnancy. They include a series of urine and serum tests.

 SUGGESTION FOR CLASSROOM ACTIVITIES

- Invite a laboratory technologist skilled in performing pregnancy tests to describe the most common pregnancy tests used to diagnose pregnancy in your community.

 SUGGESTION FOR CLINICAL ACTIVITIES

- Allow students to observe how urine and serum tests are done at a lab in a prenatal clinic to diagnose pregnancy.

LEARNING OUTCOME 4

Address the emotional and psychologic changes that commonly occur in a woman, her partner, and her family during pregnancy when providing nursing care.

Concepts for Lecture

1. During pregnancy, the expectant mother faces significant changes and must deal with major psychosocial adjustments.
2. During pregnancy, the expectant father also has to go through a period of psychosocial adjustments.
3. Pregnancy can be considered a maturational crisis since it is a common event in the normal growth and development of the family.

 POWERPOINT SLIDES 44–50

 SUGGESTIONS FOR CLASSROOM ACTIVITIES

- For classroom activity, go to *mynursingkit.com*. Assign them to locate and complete activities on prenatal education.
- Discuss Reva Rubin's four maternal tasks in pregnancy and related nursing care to help the client achieve those tasks.

 SUGGESTION FOR CLINICAL ACTIVITIES

- Assign students to a prenatal clinic. Allow them to conduct surveys on newly diagnosed pregnant couples. The surveys should focus on how the mother and father feel about the pregnancy. If grandparents and siblings are present, recommend that the survey include them. At the end of the clinical day at postclinical conference, allow students to discuss their findings in terms of the emotional and psychological changes in the family during pregnancy.

LEARNING OUTCOME 5

Recognize cultural factors that may influence a family's response to pregnancy in the provision of nursing care.

Concepts for Lecture

1. Cultural assessment is an important aspect of prenatal care.
2. Cultural assessment will help to identify cultural factors that will impact the family's plan for the pregnancy.

 POWERPOINT SLIDES 51–54

 SUGGESTION FOR CLASSROOM ACTIVITIES

- Conduct a class review of "Complementary Care: Herbs During Pregnancy." Allow students to discuss the implications of the use of herbs during pregnancy.

 SUGGESTION FOR CLINICAL ACTIVITIES

- Assign students to care for clients from multicultural backgrounds. Ask students to find out about birth practices specific to each client's culture.

GENERAL CHAPTER CONSIDERATIONS

1. Have students study and learn key terms listed at beginning of chapter.
2. Have students complete end-of-chapter exercises either in their book or on the MyNursingKit website.
3. Use the Classroom Response Questions provided in PowerPoint to assess students prior to lecture.

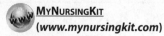

MYNURSINGKIT
(*www.mynursingkit.com*)

- NCLEX RN® review questions
- Case Studies
- Care Plans
- Critical Concept Review
- Thinking Critically
- Weblinks
- Weblink applications
- Nursing Tools
- Audio Glossary
- Images and Tables Library

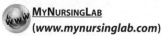

MYNURSINGLAB
(*www.mynursinglab.com*)

- Knowledge Quick Check
- Pre/Posttests
- Customized study plans
- Images and Tables Library
- *Separate purchase*

CLINICAL SKILLS MANUAL

- *Separate purchase*

PEARSON ETEXT

- Students can search, highlight, take notes, and more all in electronic format
- *Separate purchase*

TESTBANK

CHAPTER 10
ANTEPARTAL NURSING ASSESSMENT

LEARNING OUTCOME 1

Use information provided on a prenatal history to identify risk factors for the mother and/or fetus.

Concepts for Lecture

1. The history is essentially a screening tool to identify factors that may place the mother or fetus at risk during the pregnancy. Refer to Table 10-1.

POWERPOINT SLIDES 21–33

Table 10–1. Prenatal high-risk factors

SUGGESTION FOR CLASSROOM ACTIVITIES

- At the end of the lecture select two students. One student will play the role of a pregnant client. The other will obtain a complete comprehensive prenatal history based on the information obtained in the lecture and textbook from the "pregnant client." The other students will observe and critique the process. Encourage students to review resources on *mynursingkit.com*

SUGGESTION FOR CLINICAL ACTIVITIES

- Arrange to have students work with a healthcare provider at a prenatal clinic. Allow them to observe and participate in the history-taking process during an initial visit. Encourage students to also participate and observe subsequent prenatal visits. At the end of the clinical allow them to compare and contrast the essential elements of both types of visits.

LEARNING OUTCOME 2

Define common obstetric terminology found in the history of maternity clients.

Concepts for Lecture

1. See PowerPoint Slides 34–43 for a list of terms that are used in recording the history of maternity clients.

POWERPOINT SLIDES 34–43

Figure 10–1. TPAL

SUGGESTION FOR CLASSROOM ACTIVITIES

- Present the class with a list of pregnancy histories using the obstetrical terms. Have them describe in narrative what the obstetrical terms mean in the history.

SUGGESTION FOR CLINICAL ACTIVITIES

- On the clinical unit have students review pregnancy histories of the women who have given birth. Discuss the findings in postconference.

Learning Outcome 3

Consider risk factors related to the father's health that are generally recorded on the prenatal record in assessing risk factors for the mother and/or fetus.

Concepts for Lecture

1. Information about the father is also documented on the prenatal record. This information will assist in the identification of risk factors.

PowerPoint Slides 44–46

Suggestion for Classroom Activities

- Present several case studies to the class, each involving a pregnant couple. In each situation have a significant factor related to the father— a genetic disease in his family history, a history of cocaine use, an Rh positive blood type, a history of domestic violence, or others. Ask students to evaluate the potential impact of this factor on the pregnancy and future of the couple and child.

Suggestion for Clinical Activities

- Allow students to continue to shadow a prenatal healthcare provider during initial prenatal visits and subsequent visits. Assign students to generate a list of risk factors for each client and baby seen based on the prenatal history of both parents.

Learning Outcome 4

Evaluate those areas of the initial assessment that reflect the psychosocial and cultural factors related to a woman's pregnancy.

Concepts for Lecture

1. The prenatal assessment holistically focuses on the woman by considering cultural and psychosocial factors that influence her health.

PowerPoint Slides 47–51

Suggestion for Classroom Activities

- Invite a healthcare provider from a different culture to discuss prenatal care in the context of the health provider's culture. Recommend that students review "Developing Cultural Competence: Using Cultural Information Effectively."

Suggestion for Clinical Activities

- Rotate students to a prenatal clinic that serves a diverse group of clients. Recommend that students interact with clients and obtain information about the individual client's diet, religion, language, and customs surrounding pregnancy and childbirth. Allow students to discuss their findings.

Learning Outcome 5

Predict the normal physiologic changes a nurse would expect to find when performing a physical assessment of a pregnant woman.

Concepts for Lecture

1. During a physical assessment, several normal physiological changes can be identified. Refer to Assessment Guides: "Initial Prenatal Assessment" and "Subsequent Prenatal Assessment."

PowerPoint Slides 52–58

Suggestion for Classroom Activities

- Provide drawings of the pregnant female anatomy. Divide students into groups. Assign a body system to individual groups. Group members will highlight the body system they have been assigned and make a list of all the normal physiological changes that may be assessed during a prenatal visit.

SUGGESTION FOR CLINICAL ACTIVITIES

• Allow students to accompany healthcare providers performing physical assessments on pregnant females. With the help of the healthcare provider, they should try to identify some of the normal assessment findings.

LEARNING OUTCOME 6

Calculate the estimated date of birth using the common methods.

Concepts for Lecture

1. Historically the due date has been called the estimated date of confinement (EDC), and different methods may be used to estimate the date of birth (EDB).

POWERPOINT SLIDES 59–63

Figure 10–2. EDB wheel

Figure 10–3. McDonald's method

SUGGESTION FOR CLASSROOM ACTIVITIES

• Provide expected date of birth (EDB) wheels in the classroom for student manipulation. Demonstrate the use of the wheel to calculate the expected date of delivery from the last menstrual period. List a number of LMPs and ask students to calculate the expected due dates using Nägele's rule. Review Figure 10-3 and demonstrate McDonald's Method to assess fundal height.

SUGGESTION FOR CLINICAL ACTIVITIES

• At a prenatal clinic or antepartum unit, allow students to practice using the wheel and Nägele's rule to calculate the EDB using the last menstrual period. Ask them to identify any differences in the expected date of delivery obtained from using the wheel and Nägele's rule.

LEARNING OUTCOME 7

Describe the essential measurements that can be determined by clinical pelvimetry.

Concepts for Lecture

1. The pelvis can be measured to determine whether its size is adequate for a vaginal birth.

POWERPOINT SLIDES 64–70

Figure 10–5. Manual measurement of inlet and outlet

Figure 10–6. Use of a closed fist to measure the outlet

SUGGESTION FOR CLASSROOM ACTIVITIES

• Bring a pelvic model to the class. Demonstrate the measurements of the pelvic inlet and outlet. Let the students practice performing those measurements.

SUGGESTION FOR CLINICAL ACTIVITIES

• Assign students to shadow a prenatal healthcare provider during measurements of the pelvis of the pregnant female. If permissible, allow them to also participate in that activity. At the end of clinical conference, students may discuss their findings and observations.

LEARNING OUTCOME 8

Consider the results of the major screening tests used during the prenatal period in the assessment of the prenatal client.

Concepts for Lecture

1. Screening tests are used in identifying risk factors and potential complications.
2. Basic screening tests such as Pap smear, urinalysis, a complete blood count, hemoglobin, Rubella titer, ABO and Rh typing, and a hepatitis screen, tests for syphilis, and gonorrhea.
3. Urine culture at 12–16 weeks.
4. Other tests that may be indicated or are offered include drug screen, HIV testing, sickle cell screen, cystic fibrosis screen, screening for chromosomal anomalies, and neural tube defects.
5. 1-hr 50 g GTT at 24–28 weeks.
6. Rectal and vaginal swabs for group B strep.

LEARNING OUTCOME 9

Assess the prenatal client for any of the danger signs of pregnancy.

Concepts for Lecture

1. It is important to identify early signs of anemia, pulmonary, and cardiovascular problems for early treatment and prevention of complications.
2. Other signs may indicate problems with other body systems.

LEARNING OUTCOME 10

Relate the components of the subsequent prenatal history and assessment to the progress of pregnancy and the nursing care of the prenatal client.

Concepts for Lecture

1. At each visit the woman will be assessed for vital signs, weight gain, blood tests, etc.

POWERPOINT SLIDES 71–74

SUGGESTION FOR CLASSROOM ACTIVITIES

- Have students develop a timeline for prenatal visits and the assessments and teaching appropriate at each visit.

SUGGESTION FOR CLINICAL ACTIVITIES

- Have students attend a prenatal clinic and teach pregnant women about the assessments and care they receive at that visit, and about screening tests that will be performed at their next visit.

POWERPOINT SLIDES 75–77

Table 10–2. Danger signs in pregnancy

SUGGESTION FOR CLASSROOM ACTIVITIES

- Divide students into two groups. Let one group of students use note cards to list about four danger signs. Members of the other group will list the possible causes of four danger signs on note cards. Allow students to match note cards, signs with possible causes. Recommend they utilize Table 10-2 for this exercise.

SUGGESTION FOR CLINICAL ACTIVITIES

- Rotate students to a high-risk prenatal clinic or antepartum unit. Allow them to work with prenatal healthcare providers and collect subjective and objective data to formulate care plans to address danger signs identified in the clients they are caring for.

POWERPOINT SLIDES 78–80

GENERAL CHAPTER CONSIDERATIONS

1. Have students study and learn key terms listed at beginning of chapter.
2. Have students complete end-of-chapter exercises either in their book or on the MyNursingKit website.
3. Use the Classroom Response Questions provided in PowerPoint to assess students prior to lecture.

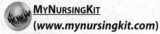

MYNURSINGKIT
(www.mynursingkit.com)

- NCLEX RN® review questions
- Case Studies
- Care Plans
- Critical Concept Review
- Thinking Critically
- Weblinks
- Weblink applications
- Nursing Tools
- Audio Glossary
- Images and Tables Library

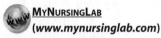

MYNURSINGLAB
(www.mynursinglab.com)

- Knowledge Quick Check
- Pre/Posttests
- Customized study plans
- Images and Tables Library
- *Separate purchase*

CLINICAL SKILLS MANUAL

- *Separate purchase*

PEARSON ETEXT

- Students can search, highlight, take notes, and more all in electronic format
- *Separate purchase*

TESTBANK

Chapter 11
The Expectant Family: Needs and Care

Learning Outcome 1

Determine the most appropriate nursing care to help maintain the well-being of the expectant father and siblings during a family's pregnancy.

Concepts for Lecture

1. Anticipatory guidance of the expectant father, if he is involved in the pregnancy, is a necessary part of any plan of care.
2. Children may feel less neglected and more secure if they know that their parents are willing to help with their anger and aggressiveness.

POWERPOINT SLIDES 20–25

Figure 11–1. The Empathy Belly® is a pregnancy simulator that allows men and women to experience some of the symptoms of pregnancy

Figure 11–5. Leg cramp relief

SUGGESTION FOR CLASSROOM ACTIVITIES

- Invite a certified nurse-midwife or a childbirth specialist to talk to your class about strategies that they as health care providers have utilized to care for childbearing families during a pregnancy.

SUGGESTION FOR CLINICAL ACTIVITIES

- Assign students to attend a childbirth class. Observe the interactions between the couples and outline the information presented during the childbirth class. Compare the information provided with the information presented in lecture format and outlined in the book. Allow students to identify similarities and new information.

Learning Outcome 2

Recognize the causes of the common discomforts of pregnancy in each of the three trimesters.

Concepts for Lecture

1. The common discomforts of pregnancy result from physiologic and anatomic changes and are fairly specific to each of the three trimesters.

POWERPOINT SLIDES 26–33

SUGGESTION FOR CLASSROOM ACTIVITIES

- For each discomfort of pregnancy ask students to develop a nursing diagnosis and expected outcome.

SUGGESTION FOR CLINICAL ACTIVITIES

- Arrange for clinical rotation at a prenatal clinic or antepartum unit. Ask students to develop teaching plans or brochures on selected discomforts of pregnancy, then ask students to review the plan with their assigned client.

Learning Outcome 3

Determine appropriate relief measures and interventions to alleviate the common discomforts of pregnancy.

Concepts for Lecture

1. Appropriate relief measures are available to deal with the common discomforts associated with pregnancy. Refer to "Complementary Care: Ginger for Morning Sickness" and Table 11-2.

PowerPoint Slides 34–46

Figure 11–2. Morning sickness relief

Figure 11–3. Relief from varicose veins

Figure 11–4. Body mechanics in pregnancy

Figure 11–8. Position for relaxation and rest as pregnancy progresses

Table 11–2. Self-care measures for common discomforts of pregnancy

Suggestion for Classroom Activities

- Divide students into two groups. Assign group A to write problems related to pregnancy on individual note cards. Then, assign group B to write treatment options on individual note cards. Place all the note cards at a central location. Allow students to match note cards, problem to treatment options. Assign students to complete the Critical Thinking in Action activity for homework.

Suggestion for Clinical Activities

- Schedule students' clinical at a prenatal clinic to work with a nurse practitioner or certified nurse-midwife. Instruct students to document all clients' complaints associated with pregnancy and the treatments recommended by the advanced-practice nurse. Allow for discussion of findings during postclinical conference.

Learning Outcome 4

Determine self-care measures that a pregnant woman can take to maintain and promote her well-being during pregnancy.

Concepts for Lecture

1. Many caregivers encourage pregnant women to monitor their unborn child's well-being by regularly assessing fetal activity beginning at 28 weeks' gestation.
2. Whether the pregnant woman plans to bottle- or breastfeed her infant, support of the breasts is important to promote comfort, retain breast shape, and prevent back strain.
3. Information about several other factors has to be considered to maintain a healthy pregnancy and facilitate maternal well-being. Refer to Table 11-2.

PowerPoint Slides 47–62

Figure 11–6. Fetal movement assessment method: the Cardiff Count-to-Ten scoring card (adaptation)

Figure 11–9. The pelvic tilt

Figure 11–10. Kegel exercises

Table 11–2. Self-care measures for common discomforts of pregnancy

Suggestion for Classroom Activities

- Using role play strategies to have students teach each other pelvic tilt and Kegel exercises.

- Schedule students to work with advanced practice nurses providing prenatal care. Let the students focus on the self-care instructions that these nurses provide for their clients.

POWERPOINT SLIDES 63–66

SUGGESTION FOR CLASSROOM ACTIVITIES

- Facilitate a review and discussion among students of "Teaching Highlights: Sexual Activity during Pregnancy."

SUGGESTION FOR CLINICAL ACTIVITIES

- As students continue their clinical rotation at a prenatal clinic with an advanced-practice nurse, recommend that they pay attention and record strategies utilized by the advanced-practice nurses when they engage in providing information about sexual activity during pregnancy to clients.

LEARNING OUTCOME 5

Address the concerns that an expectant couple might have about sexual activity.

Concepts for Lecture

1. Couples usually have many questions and concerns about sexual activity during pregnancy. They should be provided with accurate information about sexual activity during pregnancy. Refer to "Teaching Highlights: Sexual Activity during Pregnancy."

LEARNING OUTCOME 6

Relate the medical risks and special concerns of the older expectant woman and her partner to the managing nursing care indicated in providing care for this population.

Concepts for Lecture

1. There are medical risks associated with pregnancy after age 35.
2. There are also special concerns associated with pregnancy after age 35.

POWERPOINT SLIDES 67–71

Figure 11–11. For many older couples, the decision to have a child may be very rewarding

SUGGESTION FOR CLASSROOM ACTIVITIES

- Invite an older couple to share their experiences about their pregnancy with your students, including their physical and emotional responses, their concerns related to their age, the labor and delivery process, and their adjustment to parenthood.

SUGGESTION FOR CLINICAL ACTIVITIES

- Assign students to a prenatal clinic or doctor's office. Allow them to shadow a prenatal provider caring for mothers over age 35. Allow students to interview clients and inquire about the client's experiences during the pregnancy.

GENERAL CHAPTER CONSIDERATIONS

1. Have students study and learn key terms listed at beginning of chapter.
2. Have students complete end-of-chapter exercises either in their book or on the MyNursingKit website.
3. Use the Classroom Response Questions provided in PowerPoint to assess students prior to lecture.

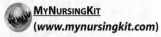

MYNURSINGKIT (*www.mynursingkit.com*)

- NCLEX RN® review questions
- Case Studies
- Care Plans
- Critical Concept Review
- Thinking Critically
- Weblinks
- Weblink applications
- Nursing Tools
- Audio Glossary
- Images and Tables Library

MYNURSINGLAB (*www.mynursinglab.com*)

- Knowledge Quick Check
- Pre/Posttests
- Customized study plans
- Images and Tables Library
- *Separate purchase*

CLINICAL SKILLS MANUAL

- *Separate purchase*

PEARSON ETEXT

- Students can search, highlight, take notes, and more all in electronic format
- *Separate purchase*

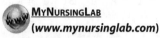

TESTBANK

Chapter 12
Maternal Nutrition

Learning Outcome 1

Consider the recommended levels of weight gain during pregnancy when providing nursing care for pregnant women.

Concepts for Lecture

1. Maternal weight gain is an important factor in fetal growth and infant birth weight.

PowerPoint Slides 20–23

Suggestion for Classroom Activities

- Review the needs of an obese pregnant client. Ask each student to develop a priority nursing diagnosis and expected outcome for the pregnant client who is obese.

Suggestion for Clinical Activities

- During clinical rotation at the prenatal clinic, assign students to participate in weighing pregnant females. Ask them to note the weight gained for each client weighed. Compare that weight to the recommended weight gain and note any deviations. Allow students to discuss their findings at the end of clinical conference.

Learning Outcome 2

Recognize the significance of specific nutrients in the diet of the pregnant woman.

Concepts for Lecture

1. The RDA for almost all nutrients increases during pregnancy, although the amount of increase varies with each nutrient. These increases reflect the additional requirements of both the mother and the developing fetus.

PowerPoint Slides 24–28

Suggestion for Classroom Activities

- Allow students to work in groups and develop a breakfast, lunch, and dinner menu high in folic acid for a woman of childbearing age.

Suggestion for Clinical Activities

- Assign students to develop a teaching plan with objectives for a pregnant mother who is experiencing anemia during pregnancy.

Learning Outcome 3

Compare nutritional needs during pregnancy, the postpartum period, and lactation with nonpregnant requirements.

Concepts for Lecture

1. During pregnancy and lactation, nutritional requirements increase significantly from nonpregnant requirements. Refer to Table 12-1.

PowerPoint Slides 29–38

Figure 12–1. MyPyramid food guide

Figure 12–4. Nutritional questionnaire

Table 12–1. Daily food plan for pregnancy and lactation

SUGGESTIONS FOR CLASSROOM ACTIVITIES

- Allow students to make a list of foods that are rich in all the nutrients outlined in the lecture.
- Provide a sample meal plan for a nonpregnant client. Have students divide into two groups. Each group will adapt the meal plan to meet the additional calorie requirements for the pregnant mother and the breastfeeding mother. Ensure that the additional needs for carbohydrates, proteins, and minerals are reflected in the meal plan.

SUGGESTION FOR CLINICAL ACTIVITIES

- Ask students to use Figure 12–4 as a guide to obtaining a diet history from a pregnant female in the prenatal unit or the antepartum unit. After obtaining the information, allow students to analyze the information based on the recommended pyramid guide.

LEARNING OUTCOME 4

Plan adequate prenatal vegetarian diets based on the nutritional requirements of pregnancy.

Concepts for Lecture

1. The expectant woman who is vegetarian must eat the proper combination of foods to obtain adequate nutrients.

POWERPOINT SLIDES 39–43

Figure 12–2. The vegetarian food pyramid

Table 12–2. Vegetarian food groups

SUGGESTION FOR CLASSROOM ACTIVITIES

- Discuss various vegetarian diets. Have students divide in groups to discuss the "Thinking Critically" scenario. Be sure to discuss the need for vitamin supplementation of a pregnant client who is a vegetarian.

SUGGESTION FOR CLINICAL ACTIVITIES

- Assign students to shadow a dietician in a prenatal environment educating pregnant vegetarian clients about the recommended food choices to sustain a healthy mother and fetus.

LEARNING OUTCOME 5

Consider ways in which various physical, psychosocial, and cultural factors can affect nutritional intake and status in the nursing care management of pregnant women.

Concepts for Lecture

1. Cultural, ethnic, and religious backgrounds determine people's experiences with food and influence food preferences and habits.

POWERPOINT SLIDES 44–47

Figure 12–3. Culture and food preferences

SUGGESTION FOR CLASSROOM ACTIVITIES

- Invite a nutritionist to your class to discuss diets reflective of clients from diverse cultural backgrounds within your community and the implications for pregnancy.

SUGGESTION FOR CLINICAL ACTIVITIES

- Assign students to clients from different cultures. Allow them to obtain diet, histories from their individual clients. Allow them to review the most common food groups in the client's diet, and based on the food pyramid guide determine whether their diets are meeting the nutrition requirements for pregnancy.

POWERPOINT SLIDES 48–52

SUGGESTION FOR CLASSROOM ACTIVITIES

- Divide the class into small groups. Ask each group to list factors that interfere with the ability of the pregnant teenager to gain weight during pregnancy. Each group will develop a teaching plan for a pregnant adolescent with weight gain concerns.

SUGGESTION FOR CLINICAL ACTIVITIES

- Arrange for students to participate in weighing pregnant adolescent clients at a prenatal clinic. Allow students to compare their individual client's weight with the recommended weight gain according to gestational age for each client. Allow them to discuss their findings during a postclinical conference.

LEARNING OUTCOME 6

Compare recommendations for weight gain and nutrient intakes in the pregnant adolescent with those for the mature pregnant adult.

Concepts for Lecture

1. Many factors that affect the weight gain of the adolescent during pregnancy need to be assessed in order to facilitate early intervention.
2. Nutritional care of the pregnant adolescent is of particular concern to healthcare professionals.

POWERPOINT SLIDES 53–57

SUGGESTION FOR CLASSROOM ACTIVITIES

- Assign students to role-play pregnant adolescent mothers and fathers during a "mock" nutritional counseling session.

SUGGESTION FOR CLINICAL ACTIVITIES

- During clinical rotation at a prenatal clinic, assign students to work with a prenatal advanced-practice provider as she or he provides nutritional counseling for teenage pregnant females.

LEARNING OUTCOME 7

Explore basic factors a nurse should consider when offering nutritional counseling to a pregnant adolescent.

Concepts for Lecture

1. Counseling about nutrition and healthy eating practices is an important element of care for pregnant teenagers that nurses can effectively provide in a community setting.

LEARNING OUTCOME 8

Compare nutritional counseling issues for breastfeeding and formula-feeding mothers.

Concepts for Lecture

1. After birth, the formula-feeding mother's dietary requirements return to prepregnancy levels.
2. Breastfeeding mothers need an increase in nutrient intake. Refer to Table 12-1.

GENERAL CHAPTER CONSIDERATIONS

1. Have students study and learn key terms listed at beginning of chapter.
2. Have students complete end-of-chapter exercises either in their book or on the MyNursingKit website.
3. Use the Classroom Response Questions provided in PowerPoint to assess students prior to lecture.

POWERPOINT SLIDES 58–61

Table 12–1. Daily food plan for pregnancy and lactation

SUGGESTIONS FOR CLASSROOM ACTIVITIES

- Instruct students to use Table 12-1 to develop a meal plan for a lactating female.
- Display various commercial formulas and have students read the ingredients for each formula.

SUGGESTIONS FOR CLINICAL ACTIVITIES

- Rotate students through a WIC clinic or ask them to attend a breastfeeding class.
- Allow students to observe a nutritionist developing meal plans for lactating females in a clinic setting.

MYNURSINGKIT
(*www.mynursingkit.com*)

- NCLEX RN® review questions
- Case Studies
- Care Plans
- Critical Concept Review
- Thinking Critically
- Weblinks
- Weblink applications
- Nursing Tools
- Audio Glossary
- Images and Tables Library

MYNURSINGLAB
(*www.mynursinglab.com*)

- Knowledge Quick Check
- Pre/Posttests
- Customized study plans
- Images and Tables Library
- *Separate purchase*

CLINICAL SKILLS MANUAL

- *Separate purchase*

PEARSON eTEXT

- Students can search, highlight, take notes, and more all in electronic format.
- *Separate purchase*

TESTBANK

CHAPTER 13
ADOLESCENT PREGNANCY

LEARNING OUTCOME 1

Recognize the scope of the problem and the impact of adolescent pregnancy.

Concepts for Lecture

1. Adolescents progress through three stages of psychosocial development. Refer to Table 13-1 and Table 13-2.
2. More than half the teens that become pregnant give birth and keep their babies. Very few adolescents give up their babies for adoption.

 POWERPOINT SLIDES 16–19

Table 13–1. Initial reaction to awareness of pregnancy

Table 13–2. The early adolescent's response to the developmental tasks of pregnancy

 SUGGESTION FOR CLASSROOM ACTIVITIES

- Facilitate student access to the Adolescent Pregnancy web links to obtain additional information about the prevalence of adolescent pregnancy in the United States and the strategies that are being utilized to decrease the incidence of teenage pregnancies.

 SUGGESTION FOR CLINICAL ACTIVITIES

- Have each student examine local and state statistics regarding teen pregnancy. Assign students to care for a pregnant adolescent.

LEARNING OUTCOME 2

Summarize factors contributing to adolescent pregnancy in the nursing care management of this population.

Concepts for Lecture

1. Many factors contribute to teenage pregnancies.

 POWERPOINT SLIDES 20–23

 SUGGESTION FOR CLASSROOM ACTIVITIES

- Assign students to write a paper about the factors that contribute to teen pregnancy in their community or state. Ask them to include information about the prevalence based on ethnic background and race. Allow students to present the information in the classroom.

 SUGGESTION FOR CLINICAL ACTIVITIES

- Schedule students to prenatal childbirth classes for pregnant teens. Instruct students to make a list of the strategies utilized by the presenter to engage the pregnant teens.

LEARNING OUTCOME 3

Assess the physical, psychologic, and sociologic risks a pregnant adolescent faces.

Concepts for Lecture

1. Unfortunately, adolescents typically begin prenatal care later in pregnancy than any other age group, which places them at risk for physical problems.
2. Teens also face psychosocial risks during pregnancy.

POWERPOINT SLIDES 24–28

SUGGESTION FOR CLASSROOM ACTIVITIES

- Place emphasis on how developmental tasks are interrupted by a pregnancy during adolescence. Ask students how the nurse can assist the pregnant adolescent and her family in meeting the developmental tasks.

SUGGESTION FOR CLINICAL ACTIVITIES

- Allow students to utilize data on prenatal records to generate a list of physical and psychosocial risks for individual clients at a prenatal pregnant teen clinic.

LEARNING OUTCOME 4

Delineate the characteristics of the fathers of children of adolescent mothers.

Concepts for Lecture

1. There are characteristic features associated with fathers of children of adolescent mothers.

POWERPOINT SLIDES 29–32

SUGGESTION FOR CLASSROOM ACTIVITIES

- Open a class discussion about fathers of babies by adolescent mothers and their involvement in the pregnancy. Ask students to state whether or not they support an active role for the father. Allow students to state reasons for their answers.

SUGGESTION FOR CLINICAL ACTIVITIES

- Suggest that students identify partners of adolescent pregnant females in the teen clinic and observe their involvement in childbirth classes or prenatal visits.

LEARNING OUTCOME 5

Discuss the range of reactions of the adolescent's family and social network to her pregnancy.

Concepts for Lecture

1. The family and social network experience a range of reactions toward an adolescent pregnancy.

POWERPOINT SLIDES 33–36

SUGGESTION FOR CLASSROOM ACTIVITIES

- At the end of the lecture allow students to review and complete the "Thinking Critically" activity and discuss their answers.

SUGGESTION FOR CLINICAL ACTIVITIES

- At the teen clinic, allow students with the guidance of the instructor or preceptor to review prenatal records of adolescent clients and conduct interviews. Instruct students to review data collected and formulate an individual, psychosocial nursing diagnosis.

Learning Outcome 6

Formulate a plan of care to meet the needs of a pregnant adolescent.

Concepts for Lecture

1. It is necessary to set goals for prenatal classes when preparing to meet the health needs of the pregnant adolescent.
2. The pregnant adolescent has the same care needs as any pregnant woman.
3. The adolescent's mother is often present during the teen's labor and birth. The father of the baby may also be involved.
4. During the postpartum period, most teens do not foresee that they will become sexually active in the near future.

Learning Outcome 7

Explore successful community approaches to prevention of adolescent pregnancy.

Concepts for Lecture

1. Effective adolescent pregnancy prevention programs are long-term and intensive.

PowerPoint Slides 37–48

Figure 13–1. Birth rates for teenagers by age: United States, final 1980–2006 and preliminary 2007

Figure 13–2. Promoting a sense of understanding and control

Suggestion for Classroom Activities

- Ask students to place in order of priority the discharge teaching needed by an adolescent mother.

Suggestion for Clinical Activities

- In clinical conference, discuss the nursing needs of the pregnant adolescent and the role of the support people.

PowerPoint Slides 49–52

Suggestion for Classroom Activities

- Assign students to prepare a presentation outlining all the adolescent pregnancy prevention programs that are available in their local community. Suggest they work in small groups. Allow students to present the information in the classroom.

Suggestion for Clinical Activities

- Assign students to spend four or more hours at a community organization that works to prevent adolescent pregnancies. Instruct students to write a paper detailing the strategies utilized by the organization to prevent teenage pregnancy.

GENERAL CHAPTER CONSIDERATIONS

1. Have students study and learn key terms listed at beginning of chapter.
2. Have students complete end-of-chapter exercises either in their book or on the MyNursingKit website.
3. Use the Classroom Response Questions provided in PowerPoint to assess students prior to lecture.

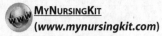

MyNursingKit
(*www.mynursingkit.com*)

- NCLEX RN® review questions
- Case Studies
- Care Plans
- Critical Concept Review
- Thinking Critically
- Weblinks
- Weblink applications
- Nursing Tools
- Audio Glossary
- Images and Tables Library

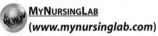

MyNursingLab
(*www.mynursinglab.com*)

- Knowledge Quick Check
- Pre/Posttests
- Customized study plans
- Images and Tables Library
- *Separate purchase*

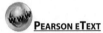

CLINICAL SKILLS MANUAL

- *Separate purchase*

PEARSON eTEXT

- Students can search, highlight, take notes, and more all in electronic format
- *Separate purchase*

TESTBANK

Chapter 14
Assessment of Fetal Well-Being

Learning Outcome 1

Identify pertinent information to be discussed with the woman regarding her own assessment of fetal activity and methods of recording fetal activity.

Concepts for Lecture

1. Clinicians now generally agree that vigorous fetal activity provides reassurance of fetal well-being.
2. The expectant mother's perception of fetal movements and her commitment to completing a fetal movement record may vary.

Learning Outcome 2

Describe the methods, clinical applications, and results of ultrasound in the nursing care management of the pregnant woman.

Concepts for Lecture

1. Valuable information about the fetus may be obtained from ultrasound testing.

 PowerPoint Slides 21–23

 Suggestion for Classroom Activities

- Assign students to prepare a teaching plan for instructing pregnant clients how to monitor and record fetal activity. Review signs and symptoms of compromised fetal activity as well as when the client should call the healthcare provider.

 Suggestion for Clinical Activities

- Allow students to engage in teaching pregnant clients about the monitoring and recording of fetal activity in a prenatal environment. Review Skill 2–8: Assessment of Fetal Well-Being: Biophysical Profile (BPP) in the *Clinical Skills Manual*.

 PowerPoint Slides 24–30

Figure 14–1. Ultrasound scanning permits visualization of the fetus in utero

Figure 14–2. Ultrasound of fetal face

 Suggestion for Classroom Activities

- Compare and contrast transabdominal and transvaginal ultrasound techniques. Highlight preprocedure and postprocedure nursing care.

Suggestion for Clinical Activities

- Assign students to an antenatal testing clinic that also performs prenatal ultrasounds. The aim of this experience is for students to observe the responsibilities of the nurse before, during, and after the ultrasound of a pregnant client.

LEARNING OUTCOME 3

Describe the use, procedure, information obtained, and nursing considerations for Doppler velocimetry, nonstress test, contraction stress test, and biophysical profile test.

Concepts for Lecture

1. Doppler blood flow studies are used to assess placental function and sufficiency.
2. A nonstress test is based on the knowledge that the FHR normally increases in response to fetal activity and to sound stimulation.
3. Biophysical profile is a combination of an ultrasound and a nonstress test used to assess fetal well-being.
4. A contraction stress test evaluates respiratory function of the placenta.

 POWERPOINT SLIDES 31–48

Figure 14–5. Example of a reactive nonstress test (NST)

Figure 14–6. Example of a nonreactive NST

Figure 14–7. NST management scheme

Figure 14–8. Example of a positive contraction stress test (CST)

Table 14–3. Nonstress test

Table 14–4. Criteria for biophysical profile scoring

Table 14–5. Contraction stress test

 SUGGESTION FOR CLASSROOM ACTIVITIES

- Ask students to compare and discuss nursing care and patient teaching for the following procedures: Doppler velocimetry, nonstress test, contraction stress test, and biophysical profile tests. End the lecture with an in-class review of Tables 14-3, 14-4, and 14-5. Assign students to review related activities for Chapter 14 on *mynursingkit.com* for homework.

 SUGGESTION FOR CLINICAL ACTIVITIES

- Allow students to observe a contraction stress test from the preparation phase to the end of the procedure. Have them turn in a written paper describing the experience using the following headings: Indication, Definition, Client Preparation, Description of Contraction Stress Test Procedure, Postprocedure Care, Reportable Signs and Symptoms, and Significance of Contraction Stress Test.

LEARNING OUTCOME 4

Explain the use of amniocentesis as a diagnostic tool.

Concepts for Lecture

1. A number of studies can be performed on amniotic fluid to determine fetal health. See "Nursing Practice."

 POWERPOINT SLIDES 49–54

Figure 14–9. Amniocentesis

 SUGGESTION FOR CLASSROOM ACTIVITIES

- Facilitate in-class review of Skill 2–5: Assisting during Amniocentesis in the *Clinical Skills Manual*.

SUGGESTION FOR CLINICAL ACTIVITIES

- During clinical rotation at the prenatal testing clinic, allow students to observe an amniocentesis. Assign students to write a paper about the procedure utilizing the following headings: Indication, Definition, Client Preparation, Description of Amniocentesis Procedure, Post-Amniocentesis Care, Reportable Signs and Symptoms, and Significance of Amniocentesis. The paper should be based on the student's observations within the clinical area and theoretical support from the textbook.

POWERPOINT SLIDES 55–59

Table 14–6. Fetal lung maturity values

SUGGESTION FOR CLASSROOM ACTIVITIES

- Review amniotic fluid analysis and patient teaching related to test results.

SUGGESTION FOR CLINICAL ACTIVITIES

- Allow students to review their assigned clients' laboratory results from an amniocentesis test. Instruct students to utilize a diagnostic textbook and a perinatal healthcare provider (NP, CNM, MD) to assist them in the interpretation of the test results.

POWERPOINT SLIDES 60–63

Table 14–1. Summary of screening and diagnostic tests

Table 14–2. Suggested nursing approaches to pretest teaching

SUGGESTION FOR CLASSROOM ACTIVITIES

- Discuss the contents of Table 14-1 and Table 14-2 in the classroom. Invite students to participate in the discussion. Include information outlined in "Nursing Practice."

SUGGESTION FOR CLINICAL ACTIVITIES

- Instruct students to prepare a generic health-teaching plan for clients undergoing prenatal testing. Allow students to participate in teaching clients before prenatal testing under the guidance of a perinatal healthcare provider.

LEARNING OUTCOME 5

Describe the tests that can be done on amniotic fluid.

Concepts for Lecture

1. Concentrations of certain substances in amniotic fluid provide information about the health status of the fetus. Refer to "Nursing Practice."

LEARNING OUTCOME 6

Compare the advantages and disadvantages of chorionic villus sampling (CVS).

Concepts for Lecture

1. Chorionic villus sampling (CVS) involves obtaining a small sample of chorionic villi from the developing placenta. CVS is performed in some medical centers for first-trimester diagnosis of genetic, metabolic, and deoxyribonucleic acid (DNA) studies. Review "Nursing Practice" and Table 14-1.

GENERAL CHAPTER CONSIDERATIONS

1. Have students study and learn key terms listed at beginning of chapter.
2. Have students complete end-of-chapter exercises either in their book or on the MyNursingKit website.
3. Use the Classroom Response Questions provided in PowerPoint to assess students prior to lecture.

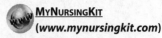

MyNursingKit (*www.mynursingkit.com*)

- NCLEX RN® review questions
- Case Studies
- Care Plans
- Critical Concept Review
- Thinking Critically
- Weblinks
- Weblink applications
- Nursing Tools
- Audio Glossary
- Images and Tables Library

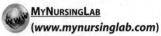

MyNursingLab (*www.mynursinglab.com*)

- Knowledge Quick Check
- Pre/Posttests
- Customized study plans
- Images and Tables Library
- *Separate purchase*

CLINICAL SKILLS MANUAL

- *Separate purchase*

PEARSON eTEXT

- Students can search, highlight, take notes, and more all in electronic format
- *Separate purchase*

TESTBANK

CHAPTER 15
PREGNANCY AT RISK: PREGESTATIONAL PROBLEMS

LEARNING OUTCOME 1

Describe the effects of alcohol and illicit drugs in the nursing care management of the childbearing woman and her fetus/newborn.

Concepts for Lecture

1. Illicit drug use during pregnancy, particularly in the first trimester, may have a negative effect on the health of the woman and the growth and development of fetus. See Table 15-1.
2. The effects of alcohol on the fetus may result in a group of signs known as fetal alcohol syndrome (FAS).

POWERPOINT SLIDES 19–33

Table 15–1. Possible effects of selected drugs of abuse or addiction on fetus and neonate

SUGGESTION FOR CLASSROOM ACTIVITIES

- Allow for in-class review of data displayed in Table 15-1. Divide the class in four groups. Each group is given the task of developing priority nursing interventions for the childbearing family impacted by illicit drug and alcohol use

SUGGESTION FOR CLINICAL ACTIVITIES

- Arrange for students to work with a prenatal provider who cares for pregnant clients with substance abuse problems in a prenatal or antepartum environment.

LEARNING OUTCOME 2

Relate the pathology and clinical treatment of diabetes mellitus in pregnancy to the implications for nursing care.

Concepts for Lecture

1. Diabetes mellitus (DM), an endocrine disorder of carbohydrate metabolism, results from inadequate production or use of insulin. States of altered carbohydrate metabolism have been classified in several ways.
2. Pregnancy can affect diabetes significantly because the physiologic changes of pregnancy can drastically alter insulin requirements.
3. The pregnancy of a woman who has diabetes carries a higher risk of complications, especially perinatal mortality and congenital anomalies.
4. Clinical therapy begins with glucose screening and aims to control blood glucose levels.

POWERPOINT SLIDES 34–47

Figure 15–1. Maternal glucose levels

Figure 15–2. Home glucose monitoring

SUGGESTIONS FOR CLASSROOM ACTIVITIES

- Allow in-class time for review of Figure 15-1 and Figure 15-2. Ask each student to develop a teaching plan for mother with gestational diabetes.
- Discuss evidence-based practice. Instruct students to review "Evidence-Based Nursing" and complete the critical thinking activity at the end.

SUGGESTION FOR CLINICAL ACTIVITIES

- Assign students to search health related Internet sites for patient teaching information related to diabetes. Have each student discuss the results of their search with the clinical group in postconference.

LEARNING OUTCOME 3

Distinguish among the types of anemia associated with pregnancy regarding signs, treatment, and implications for pregnancy.

Concepts for Lecture

1. Anemia indicates inadequate levels of hemoglobin in the blood. There are characteristic signs and symptoms associated with a diagnosis of anemia.
2. There are different types of anemia associated with pregnancy complications. Early recognition and treatment of anemia reduces pregnancy complications. Refer to Table 15-4.

POWERPOINT SLIDES 48–51

Table 15–4. Anemia and pregnancy

SUGGESTIONS FOR CLASSROOM ACTIVITIES

- Ask students to use Table 15-4 to outline the maternal and fetal risks associated with each type of anemia.
- Divide students into two groups. Have one group develop a menu that includes foods high in iron and the other group develop a menu that includes foods high in folic acid.

SUGGESTION FOR CLINICAL ACTIVITIES

- Allow students to review the hemoglobin levels of a group of clients at a prenatal clinic. Ask them to identify the clients with anemia based on hemoglobin levels. Students should be encouraged to get additional information from the prenatal chart and prenatal healthcare provider to determine the type of anemia each client was diagnosed with.

LEARNING OUTCOME 4

Describe acquired immunodeficiency syndrome (AIDS), including care of the pregnant woman who has tested positive for the human immunodeficiency virus (HIV), fetal/neonatal implications, and ramifications for the childbearing family.

Concepts for Lecture

1. Human immunodeficiency virus (HIV) infection is one of today's major health concerns. It leads to a progressive disease that ultimately results in acquired immunodeficiency syndrome.
2. Many women who are HIV positive choose to avoid pregnancy because of the risk of infecting the fetus.
3. There are established guidelines for the management of pregnant women with HIV infection. Refer to "Nursing Care Plan: The Woman with HIV Infection."

POWERPOINT SLIDES 52–63

SUGGESTION FOR CLASSROOM ACTIVITIES

- Instruct students to review "Nursing Care Plan: The Woman with HIV Infection."

VIDEO CLIPS

Zidovudine

SUGGESTION FOR CLINICAL ACTIVITIES

- Assign students to a prenatal HIV clinic. Request that students review the prenatal records of their individual clients before participating in the care of the client. Instruct them to utilize the subjective and objective data collected to outline a nursing care plan for each client.

LEARNING OUTCOME 5

Explain the effects of various heart disorders on pregnancy, including implications for nursing care management in the antepartum, intrapartum, and postpartum periods.

Concepts for Lecture

1. The woman with heart disease has decreased cardiac reserve, making it more difficult for her heart to handle the higher workload of pregnancy.

POWERPOINT SLIDES 64–71

Figure 15–3. Monitoring for signs of heart failure

Table 15–5. Severity of heart disease by functional capacity

2. The pathology found in a pregnant woman with heart disease varies with the type of disorder.
3. The primary goal of clinical therapy is early diagnosis and ongoing management of the woman with cardiac disease.

LEARNING OUTCOME 6

Delineate the effects of selected pregestational medical conditions on pregnancy.

Concepts for Lecture

1. A woman with a preexisting medical condition needs to be aware of the possible impact of pregnancy on her condition, as well as the impact of her condition on the successful outcome of her pregnancy. Refer to Table 15-6.

SUGGESTION FOR CLASSROOM ACTIVITIES

• Invite a cardiologist to talk to the students about heart disease and the implications for pregnancy.

SUGGESTION FOR CLINICAL ACTIVITIES

• Arrange for students to spend some clinical time in a high-risk perinatal care unit. If possible, assist in the selection of pregnant or laboring females who have been diagnosed with cardiac disease. Each student should be paired with an experienced perinatal registered nurse. The students should focus on observing the overall clinical and nursing management of their individual clients.

POWERPOINT SLIDES 72–74

Table 15–6. Less common medical conditions and pregnancy

SUGGESTION FOR CLASSROOM ACTIVITIES

• Begin the class by talking about the most common medical conditions that may complicate a pregnancy. Utilize Table 15-6 to focus on the common conditions listed in the book.

SUGGESTION FOR CLINICAL ACTIVITIES

• Students should continue their clinical experience at the high-risk perinatal unit. Assign students to shadow registered nurses caring for pregnant clients with medical conditions. Select one student to present subjective and objective data collected on the client. Allow the other students to use the data presented to identify a list of nursing diagnosis for that client.

GENERAL CHAPTER CONSIDERATIONS

1. Have students study and learn key terms listed at beginning of chapter.
2. Have students complete end-of-chapter exercises either in their book or on the MyNursingKit website.
3. Use the Classroom Response Questions provided in PowerPoint to assess students prior to lecture.

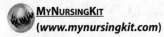

MyNursingKit
(www.mynursingkit.com)

- NCLEX RN® review questions
- Case Studies
- Care Plans
- Critical Concept Review
- Thinking Critically
- Weblinks
- Weblink applications
- Nursing Tools
- Audio Glossary
- Images and Tables Library

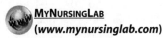

MyNursingLab
(www.mynursinglab.com)

- Knowledge Quick Check
- Pre/Posttests
- Customized study plans
- Images and Tables Library
- *Separate purchase*

CLINICAL SKILLS MANUAL

- *Separate purchase*

PEARSON eTEXT

- Students can search, highlight, take notes, and more all in electronic format
- *Separate purchase*

TESTBANK

CHAPTER 16
PREGNANCY AT RISK: GESTATIONAL PROBLEMS

LEARNING OUTCOME 1

Summarize the etiology, medical therapy, and cultural perspectives to community-based and hospital-based nursing care management of women with a bleeding problem associated with pregnancy.

Concepts for Lecture

1. During the first and second trimesters, abortion is the major cause of bleeding.
2. Other complications that may cause bleeding in the first half of pregnancy are ectopic pregnancy and gestational trophoblastic disease.
3. In the second half of pregnancy, particularly in the third trimester, the two major causes of bleeding are placenta previa and abruptio placentae.
4. The nurse has certain general responsibilities in providing nursing care for clients experiencing bleeding during pregnancy.

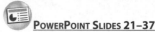

PowerPoint Slides 21–37

Figure 16–1. Types of spontaneous abortion

Figure 16–2. Hydatidiform mole

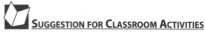

Suggestion for Classroom Activities

- Discuss nursing implications of methotrexate use with a client experiencing ectopic pregnancy.

Suggestion for Clinical Activities

- Schedule students' clinical time at a high-risk prenatal clinic or an antepartum unit. Arrange for them to care for clients diagnosed with bleeding during pregnancy along with a primary nurse. They should participate in assessment data collection. Ask them to make a list of the nursing interventions carried out or observed during their clinical rotation.

LEARNING OUTCOME 2

Describe the maternal and fetal-neonatal risks and medical therapy in the nursing care management of a woman with hyperemesis gravidarum.

Concepts for Lecture

1. Hyperemesis gravidarum, a relatively rare condition, is excessive vomiting during pregnancy.
2. Treatment of hyperemesis gravidarum is aimed at controlling vomiting and maintaining fluid and electrolyte status.
3. The nurse's role in caring for a client diagnosed with hyperemesis gravidarum is multifaceted.

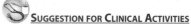

PowerPoint Slides 38–41

Suggestion for Classroom Activities

- Instruct students to make a list of nursing diagnoses that applies to a client diagnosed with hyperemesis gravidarum. Tell the students to write a minimum of two nursing interventions for each listed nursing diagnosis.

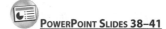

Suggestion for Clinical Activities

- Arrange for clinical rotation at an antepartum unit. Assign students to observe and participate in the care of clients diagnosed with hyperemesis gravidarum. Allow students to formulate care plans for each assigned client.

LEARNING OUTCOME 3

Describe the maternal and fetal-neonatal risks, clinical manifestations, and diagnosis in determining the nursing care management of a pregnant woman with a hypertensive disorder.

Concepts for Lecture

1. A number of hypertensive disorders can occur during pregnancy.
2. Hypertensive disorders that occur during pregnancy place the pregnant female, the fetus, or the newborn at risk for complications.
3. Clinical manifestations depend on whether the condition is mild, severe, or complicated with the occurrence of eclampsia.
4. Clinical and nursing management is dependent on the severity of the disease. See "Nursing Care Plan for a Woman with Preeclampsia" and "Drug Guide: Magnesium Sulfate."

 POWERPOINT SLIDES 42–60

Figure 16–4. Assessing clonus

Table 16–1. Deep tendon reflex rating scale

 SUGGESTION FOR CLASSROOM ACTIVITIES

- Have students divide into groups. Assign groups to develop priority nursing diagnoses for a client receiving magnesium sulfate, a client with HELLP syndrome, and a client with eclampsia.

 SUGGESTION FOR CLINICAL ACTIVITIES

- Before clinical, tell students to review "Skill 2–3: Assessing Deep Tendon Reflexes and Clonus" in the *Clinical Skills Manual.* Allow for clinical practice of deep tendon assessment and clonus at the clinical site. Review with students how to assess edema in a client with preeclampsia.

LEARNING OUTCOME 4

Relate the cause, fetal-neonatal risks, prevention, and clinical therapy to the nursing care management of the woman at risk for Rh alloimmunization.

Concepts for Lecture

1. Rh alloimmunization (sensitization), also called isoimmunization, most often occurs when an Rh-negative woman carries an Rh-positive fetus, either to term or to termination by miscarriage or induced abortion.

 POWERPOINT SLIDES 61–69

Figure 16–5. Rh alloimmunization sequence

Table 16–2. Rh alloimmunization

 SUGGESTIONS FOR CLASSROOM ACTIVITIES

- Divide the class into three groups. Have each group develop the following:
  1. Nursing implications for a client receiving Rh immune globulin.
  2. Patient teaching related to Rh Immune globulin
  3. Nursing implications of the Direct and Indirect Combs tests.

 SUGGESTION FOR CLINICAL ACTIVITIES

- Students should be allowed to participate in the screening, identification, education, and nursing management of pregnant women who have Rh-negative blood. They may do so at a prenatal clinic or an antepartum, intrapartum, or postpartum unit under the supervision of a preceptor or clinical instructor.

LEARNING OUTCOME 5

Explain the occurrence, cause, clinical treatment, and implications for the fetus or newborn in determining the nursing care management of a woman at risk for ABO incompatibility.

Concepts for Lecture

1. In most cases, ABO incompatibility is limited to type O mothers with a type A, B, or AB fetus. Unlike Rh incompatibility, no treatment exists to prevent the occurrence.

LEARNING OUTCOME 6

Examine the effects of surgical procedures in the nursing care management of the pregnant woman requiring surgery.

Concepts for Lecture

1. Elective surgery poses some risks and should be delayed until the postpartum, but essential surgery can generally be done during pregnancy.
2. Special considerations must be kept in mind whenever the surgical client is pregnant.

LEARNING OUTCOME 7

Relate the impact of trauma caused by an accident to the nursing care management of the pregnant woman or her fetus.

Concepts for Lecture

1. Trauma complicates 6% to 7% of pregnancies and is the leading nonobstetric cause of maternal death. When major blunt trauma to the mother occurs in the second or third trimester the risk of fetal loss is 40% to 50%.
2. Treatment of major injuries during pregnancy focuses initially on lifesaving measures for the woman and the fetus.

POWERPOINT SLIDES 70–73

SUGGESTION FOR CLASSROOM ACTIVITIES

- Have students search *Medlineplus.gov* for articles related to ABO incompatibility.

SUGGESTION FOR CLINICAL ACTIVITIES

- Ask each student to develop a teaching for childbearing families experiencing ABO incompatibility.

POWERPOINT SLIDES 74–78

SUGGESTION FOR CLASSROOM ACTIVITIES

- Ask students to make a list of all the physiologic changes according to body systems associated with pregnancy and for each change show how surgery may impact the physiologic status of the pregnant female. Allow guided classroom discussion.

SUGGESTION FOR CLINICAL ACTIVITIES

- Arrange for students to observe and participate in caring for pregnant clients during the preoperative, intraoperative, and postoperative phases of surgery under the guidance of a clinical instructor. Instruct students to write about the observations that they made and to identify actual or potential problems associated with their client's surgery.

POWERPOINT SLIDES 79–85

ANIMATION

Premature Labor

SUGGESTION FOR CLASSROOM ACTIVITIES

- In preparation for this lecture, assign students to obtain information about the prevalence and causes of trauma during pregnancy in their local community. Allow students to discuss their findings in the classroom. Review CPR procedures on pregnant women.

SUGGESTION FOR CLINICAL ACTIVITIES

- Arrange to have students gain clinical experience in an obstetric triage unit. Assign students to shadow a prenatal healthcare provider who evaluates pregnant clients involved in motor vehicle accidents or sustained trauma by other means. Instruct students to write a paper describing the evaluation process for each client observed.

LEARNING OUTCOME 8

Delineate the needs and care of the pregnant woman who experiences abuse.

Concepts for Lecture

1. Domestic violence, most often the intentional injury of a woman by her partner, often begins or increases during pregnancy.
2. The goals of treatment are to identify the woman at risk, to increase her decision-making abilities to decrease the risk for further abuse, and to provide a safe environment for the woman and her unborn child.

POWERPOINT SLIDES 86–92

SUGGESTION FOR CLASSROOM ACTIVITIES

- Invite a social worker to talk to the students about the incidence of spousal abuse in the local community and the strategies currently utilized in the local community to address this problem.

SUGGESTION FOR CLINICAL ACTIVITIES

- As part of the students' clinical assignment, allow them to gather information in their local community about the community resources available to pregnant females facing physical abuse. Students should also be allowed to spend some time at a shelter for pregnant, abused clients. Students should focus on the services available to help pregnant, physically abused females at the shelter they have been assigned to.

LEARNING OUTCOME 9

Explain the causes, fetal-neonatal risks, and clinical therapy in the nursing care management of the pregnant woman with a perinatal infection affecting the fetus

Concepts for Lecture

1. Infections acquired during pregnancy may have an impact on the fetus. Refer to Table 16-3.

POWERPOINT SLIDES 93–103

Table 16–3. Infections that put pregnancy at risk

SUGGESTION FOR CLASSROOM ACTIVITIES

- Divide students into three groups. Ask each group to single out a specific infection and develop a Care Plan for a pregnant woman with that perinatal infection

SUGGESTION FOR CLINICAL ACTIVITIES

- Assign students to an antepartum unit or prenatal clinic. Allow them to review prenatal or medical records of the clients they have been assigned to care for. They should pay particular attention to subjective and objective information including laboratory results. Instruct them to utilize the assessment data to identify clients with prenatal infections or clients at risk for prenatal infections. Allow them to make a list of possible nursing diagnoses for each of their clients.

GENERAL CHAPTER CONSIDERATIONS

1. Have students study and learn key terms listed at beginning of chapter.
2. Have students complete end-of-chapter exercises either in their book or on the MyNursingKit website.
3. Use the Classroom Response Questions provided in PowerPoint to assess students prior to lecture.

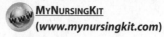 **MyNursingKit**
(*www.mynursingkit.com*)

- NCLEX RN® review questions
- Case Studies
- Care Plans
- Critical Concept Review
- Thinking Critically
- Weblinks
- Weblink applications
- Nursing Tools
- Audio Glossary
- Images and Tables Library

 MyNursingLab
(*www.mynursinglab.com*)

- Knowledge Quick Check
- Pre/Posttests
- Customized study plans
- Images and Tables Library
- *Separate purchase*

CLINICAL SKILLS MANUAL

- *Separate purchase*

 PEARSON eTEXT

- Students can search, highlight, take notes, and more all in electronic format
- *Separate purchase*

 TESTBANK

Chapter 17
Processes and Stages of Labor and Birth

Learning Outcome 1

Describe the five critical factors that influence labor in the assessment of an expectant woman's and fetus's progress in labor and birth.

Concepts for Lecture

1. Birth passage: The ability of the pelvis and cervix to accommodate the passage of the fetus.
2. Fetus: The ability of the fetus to complete the birth process.
3. Relationship between the passage and the fetus: The position of the fetus in relation to the pelvis.
4. Physiologic forces of labor: Characteristics of contractions and the effectiveness of expulsion methods.
5. Psychosocial considerations: Understanding and preparing for the childbirth experience. Amount of support from other. Present emotional status. Beliefs and values.

 PowerPoint Slides 23–38

Figures 17–1. Comparison of Caldwell-Moloy pelvic types

Figure 17–2. Superior view of the fetal skull

Figure 17–5. Fetal attitude

Figure 17–7. Process of engagement in cephalic presentation

Figure 17–8. Measuring the station of the fetal head while it is descending

Figure 17–10. Characteristics of uterine contractions

Table 17–2. Implications of pelvic type for labor and birth

 Video Clips

Fetal Lie

 Suggestions for Classroom Activities

- Demonstrate attitude, lie, and presentation with a baby doll or fetal model.
- Use a pelvis model to demonstrate station.

 Suggestion for Clinical Activities

- Ask students to discuss what factors impact fetal circulation during labor.

LEARNING OUTCOME 2

Examine an expectant woman's and fetus's response to labor based on the physiologic processes that occur during labor.

Concepts for Lecture

1. Progesterone causes relaxation of smooth muscle tissue. Estrogen causes stimulation of uterine muscle contractions. Connective tissue loosens and permits the softening, thinning, and opening of the cervix.
2. Muscles of the upper uterine segment shorten and cause the cervix to thin and flatten. Fetal body is straightened as the uterus elongates with each contraction.
3. Pressure of the fetal head causes cervical dilation. Rectum and vagina are drawn upward and forward with each contraction. During the second stage, the anus everts.

LEARNING OUTCOME 3

Assess for the premonitory signs of labor when caring for the expectant woman.

Concepts for Lecture

1. Lightening—Braxton Hicks contractions.
2. Cervical changes—bloody show.
3. Rupture of membranes—sudden burst of energy.
4. Other signs may occur prior to the onset of labor.

LEARNING OUTCOME 4

Differentiate between false and true labor.

Concepts for Lecture

1. True labor is characterized by: Contractions that occur at regular intervals and increase in duration and intensity; discomfort that begins in the back and radiates to the front of the abdomen; walking intensifies contractions; resting or relaxing in warm water does not decrease the intensity of contractions; contractions that produce cervical dilatation.

POWERPOINT SLIDES 39–42

VIDEO CLIPS
First Stage of Labor

SUGGESTIONS FOR CLASSROOM ACTIVITIES
- Discuss and demonstrate the cardinal movements of labor with a fetal model or baby doll.
- View the video "First Stage of Labor" on *mynursingkit.com*

SUGGESTION FOR CLINICAL ACTIVITIES
- Have students develop a care map on the physiology of labor and how it impacts each body system.

POWERPOINT SLIDES 43–47

ANIMATION
Rupturing Membranes

SUGGESTIONS FOR CLASSROOM ACTIVITIES
- Discuss the human needs an expectant mother has when experiencing the premonitory signs of labor. Review the animation "Rupturing Membranes" on *mynursingkit.com*
- Have students suck on Lifesavers candies and note how the candy thins and the center hole enlarges. Compare to cervical changes prior to and during labor.

SUGGESTION FOR CLINICAL ACTIVITIES
- Ask students to design a teaching plan regarding the signs and symptoms of labor. Have them teach an expectant mother and her partner at an antepartum clinic.

POWERPOINT SLIDES 48–51

Table 17–4. Comparison of true and false labor

SUGGESTION FOR CLASSROOM ACTIVITIES
- Discuss the psychological needs of an expectant mother who has experienced false labor. Have students prepare a one-page teaching pamphlet to use with prenatal clients when teaching them to differentiate between false and true labor.

2. False labor is characterized by: Irregular contractions that do not increase in duration or intensity; contractions that are lessened by walking, rest, or warm water; discomfort that is felt primarily in the abdomen; contractions that produce no effect on cervix.

LEARNING OUTCOME 5

Describe the physiologic and psychologic changes occurring in an expectant woman during each stage of labor in the nursing care management of the expectant woman.

Concepts for Lecture

1. Latent phase physiologic changes: Regular, mild contractions begin and increase in intensity and frequency; cervical effacement and dilation begins. Latent phase psychologic changes: Relief that labor has begun; high excitement with some anxiety.
2. Active phase physiologic changes: Contractions increase in intensity, frequency, and duration; cervical dilation increases from 4 to 7 cm; fetus begins to descend into the pelvis. Active phase psychologic changes: fear of loss of control; anxiety increases; possible decrease in coping skills.
3. Transition phase physiologic changes: Contractions continue to increase in intensity, duration, and frequency; cervix dilates from 8 to 10 cm; fetus descends rapidly into the birth passage; woman may experience rectal pressure; woman may experience nausea and/or vomiting. Transition phase psychologic changes: increased feelings of anxiety; irritability; eager to complete birth experience; need to have support person or nurse at bedside.
4. Second stage physiologic changes: Begins with complete cervical dilation and ends with the birth of the infant; woman pushes due to pressure of fetal head on sacral and obturator nerves; woman uses intra-abdominal pressure; perineum begins to bulge, flatten, and move anteriorly as fetus descends. Second stage psychologic changes: May feel a sense of purpose; may feel out of control, frightened, and irritable.
5. Third stage physiologic changes: Placental separation—uterus contracts and the placenta begins to separate; placental delivery—woman bears down and delivers the placenta. Physician may put slight traction on the cord to assist the delivery of the placenta. Third stage psychologic changes: Woman may feel relief at the completion of the birth; woman is usually focused on welfare of the infant and may not recognize that placental expulsion is occurring.
6. Fourth stage physiologic changes: Woman experiences increased pulse and decreased blood pressure due to redistribution of blood from uterus and blood loss; uterus remains contracted and is located between umbilicus and symphysis pubis; woman may experience a shaking chill; urine may be retained due to decreased bladder tone and possible trauma to the bladder. Fourth stage psychologic changes: May experience euphoria and energized at birth of child; may be thirsty and hungry.

SUGGESTION FOR CLINICAL ACTIVITIES
- Have students attend a childbirth class. Ask them to document what the expectant mothers learn about true and false labor.

POWERPOINT SLIDES 52–64

Table 17–5. Characteristics of labor

ANIMATION
Vaginal Birth

ANIMATION
Placenta Delivery

VIDEO CLIPS
First Stage of Labor and Transition

VIDEO CLIPS
Second Stage of Labor

VIDEO CLIPS
Third Stage of Labor

SUGGESTION FOR CLASSROOM ACTIVITIES
- In class, show the Vaginal Birth Animation from *mynursingkit.com*. Discuss the complementary therapies that may be of value to a mother during birth. Have students view the videos "Second Stage of Labor" and "Third Stage of Labor" as well as the animation "Placenta Delivery" on the *mynursingkit.com* for review.

SUGGESTIONS FOR CLINICAL ACTIVITIES
- Assign students to write a reflective journal after they have observed a vaginal delivery. Have them elaborate on the role of the nurse.
- In postconference, ask each student to develop a psychological nursing diagnosis for each stage of labor for the mother.

LEARNING OUTCOME 6

Explain the maternal systemic response to labor in the nursing care of an expectant woman.

Concepts for Lecture

1. Cardiovascular changes: Increase in cardiac output; blood pressure—rises with each contraction and may rise further with pushing; respiratory system—increase in oxygen demand and consumption. Mild respiratory acidosis usually occurs by time of birth.
2. Renal system: Increase in renin, plasma renin activity, and angiotensinogen. Edema may occur at base of bladder due to pressure of fetal head.
3. Gastrointestinal system: Gastric motility decreased. Gastric emptying is prolonged. Gastric volume remains increased—immune system and other blood values: WBC count increases. Blood glucose decreases.
4. Pain: In the first stage, it arises from dilation of cervix, stretching of lower uterine segment, pressure, and hypoxia of uterine muscle cells during contractions. In the second stage, it arises from hypoxia of contracting uterine muscle cells, distention of the vagina and perineum, and pressure. In the third stage, it arises from contractions and dilation of cervix as placenta is expelled.

LEARNING OUTCOME 7

Examine fetal responses to labor.

Concepts for Lecture

1. Labor may cause no adverse effects in the healthy fetus. Fetal heart rate may decrease as the head pushes against the cervix. Blood flow decreases to the fetus at the peak of each contraction leading to a decrease in pH. Further decrease of pH occurs during pushing due to the woman holding her breath.

 POWERPOINT SLIDES 65–72

Figure 17–14. Placental separation and expulsion

 SUGGESTION FOR CLASSROOM ACTIVITIES

- Discuss priority nursing assessments and interventions during the fourth stage of labor. Include nutritional needs of the mother at this time.

 SUGGESTION FOR CLINICAL ACTIVITIES

- Assign students to care for mothers during the fourth stage of labor. Ask them to develop one physical and one psychosocial nursing diagnosis with interventions.

 POWERPOINT SLIDES 73–75

 SUGGESTIONS FOR CLASSROOM ACTIVITIES

- Discuss the following physiologic changes in the fetus and which adverse effects can occur in each category: heart rate changes, acid-base changes in labor, hemodynamic changes, and fetal sensation.
- Place plastic figurine and rope into a balloon. Partially fill the balloon with water and seal. Have students observe the results of "contractions" on the figurine when balloon is intact, and again when fluid is released through a pinhole. Relate this rupture of membranes and effects of increased pressure on the fetal head and cord.

 SUGGESTION FOR CLINICAL ACTIVITIES

- Assign students to care for clients in a variety of labor situations, noting and comparing the influence of latent phase versus transitional or second stage contractions on fetal heart tracings. In postclinical conferences, ask students to discuss what sensations the fetus experiences during labor.

GENERAL CHAPTER CONSIDERATIONS

1. Have students study and learn key terms listed at beginning of chapter.
2. Have students complete end-of-chapter exercises either in their book or on the MyNursingKit website.
3. Use the Classroom Response Questions provided in PowerPoint to assess students prior to lecture.

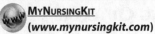

MyNursingKit
(*www.mynursingkit.com*)

- NCLEX RN® review questions
- Case Studies
- Care Plans
- Critical Concept Review
- Thinking Critically
- Weblinks
- Weblink applications
- Nursing Tools
- Audio Glossary
- Images and Tables Library

MyNursingLab
(*www.mynursinglab.com*)

- Knowledge Quick Check
- Pre/Posttests
- Customized study plans
- Images and Tables Library
- *Separate purchase*

CLINICAL SKILLS MANUAL

- *Separate purchase*

PEARSON eTEXT

- Students can search, highlight, take notes, and more all in electronic format
- *Separate purchase*

TESTBANK

CHAPTER 18
INTRAPARTAL NURSING ASSESSMENT

LEARNING OUTCOME 1

Describe a maternal assessment of the laboring woman that includes the client history, high-risk screening, and physical and psychosociocultural factors.

Concepts for Lecture

1. High-risk screening is completed to determine if there are any factors present that may be associated with a high-risk condition. See Table 18-1.
2. Maternal physical factors include vital signs, labor status, fetal status, laboratory finding. Cultural assessment includes individual beliefs and preferences. Psychosocial factors assessed include childbearing findings.

LEARNING OUTCOME 2

Evaluate the progress of labor by assessing the laboring woman's contractions, cervical dilatation, and effacement.

Concepts for Lecture

1. Assessment of contractions for frequency, strength, and intensity of contractions. See "Skill 3-5: External Electronic Fetal Monitoring" and "Skill 3-6: Internal Electronic Fetal Monitoring" in the *Clinical Skills Manual.*
2. Cervical assessment includes:
   a. Determination of cervical dilatation—from 1 cm to 10 cm.
   b. Determination of effacement—measured in percentage. Full effacement is 100%.
3. Vaginal examination assists in the evaluation of descent and status of membranes. See "Skill 3-4: Auscultating Fetal Heart Rate" in the *Clinical Skills Manual.*

 POWERPOINT SLIDES 20–33

Table 18–1. Intrapartal high-risk factors

 SUGGESTION FOR CLASSROOM ACTIVITIES

- Review maternity assessment forms with the class. Divide the class in groups. Have each group review Table 18-1 and develop a priority nursing diagnosis for each risk factor.

 SUGGESTION FOR CLINICAL ACTIVITIES

- Review maternity assessment forms with the clinical group. Have students assist with the admission of a laboring client. Have students rotate through a healthcare provider's office.

 POWERPOINT SLIDES 34–50

Figure 18–1. Woman in labor with external monitor applied

Figure 18–2. Gauging cervical dilatation

Figure 18–3. Palpating the presenting part (portion of the fetus that enters the pelvis first)

Figure 18–8. Technique for internal, direct fetal monitoring

Table 18–2. Contraction and labor progress characteristics

 SUGGESTION FOR CLASSROOM ACTIVITIES

- Discuss internal and external fetal monitoring assessment during labor. What makes assessments different? What information is learned from each type of monitoring?

 SUGGESTION FOR CLINICAL ACTIVITIES

- Show students intrauterine pressure catheter. Have students review the institution's protocol for internal fetal monitoring. Ask students to compare the protocol with their textbook.

LEARNING OUTCOME 3

Describe the steps and frequency for performing auscultation of fetal heart rate.

Concepts for Lecture

1. Vaginal examination assists in the evaluation of descent and status of membranes. See "Skill 3-4: Auscultating Fetal Heart Rate" in the *Clinical Skills Manual*.

LEARNING OUTCOME 4

Delineate the procedure for performing Leopold's maneuvers and the information that can be obtained.

Concepts for Lecture

1. Leopold's maneuvers evaluate the position, presentation, and lie of the fetus by palpation of the woman's abdomen. The woman empties her bladder and lies on her back with her knees flexed. The practitioner palpates the abdomen gently but deeply using the palms of the hands. One hand is held steady while the other explores one side of the abdomen, then the action of the hands is switched.

LEARNING OUTCOME 5

Distinguish between baseline and periodic changes in fetal heart rate monitoring, and the appearance and significance of each.

Concepts for Lecture

1. Baseline rate refers to the average fetal heart rate observed during a 10-minute period of monitoring. Normal rate is 110-160 bpm. Baseline changes include bradycardia, tachycardia, and variability.
2. Periodic changes include accelerations, decelerations, and variability.

POWERPOINT SLIDES 51–58

Figure 18–6. Location of FHR in relation to the more commonly seen fetal positions

SUGGESTION FOR CLASSROOM ACTIVITIES

- Discuss routine use of EFM, recent studies about its efficacy, and its role in nursing resource allocation. Talk about evidence-based practice. Have students review "Skills 3-4: Auscultating Fetal Heart Rate" and "3-5: Electronic Fetal Monitoring" in the *Clinical Skills Manual*.

SUGGESTION FOR CLINICAL ACTIVITIES

- Have students practice auscultation FHT by Doppler, fetoscope (where available), and EFM in the clinical laboratory.

POWERPOINT SLIDES 59–65

Figure 18–5. Leopold's maneuvers for determining fetal position and presentation

SUGGESTION FOR CLASSROOM ACTIVITIES

- Include a variety of monitor strips. Discuss rate, periodic patterns, and variability. Have students review "Skill 3-3: Performing Leopold's Maneuvers" in the *Clinical Skills Manual*.

SUGGESTION FOR CLINICAL ACTIVITIES

- Assign students to an antepartum clinic where they can observe and perform Leopold's maneuvers on pregnant clients. If possible, have students use multiparous women or women with epidurals, as it is sometimes easier to palpate small parts due to frequently weaker or more relaxed abdominal muscles.

POWERPOINT SLIDES 66–74

SUGGESTION FOR CLASSROOM ACTIVITIES

- Review a nonreassuring tracing and explore the causes, nursing interventions, and outcomes.

SUGGESTION FOR CLINICAL ACTIVITIES

- Demonstrate use of the Doppler and the fetoscope. Then, assign students to care for laboring clients with electronic fetal monitoring.

LEARNING OUTCOME 6

Evaluate fetal heart rate tracings using a systematic approach.

Concepts for Lecture

1. Evaluate the uterine contraction pattern.
2. Determine the baseline fetal heart rate; determine fetal heart rate variability; and determine if a sinusoidal pattern is present.
3. Determine if there are periodic changes.

POWERPOINT SLIDES 75–78

SUGGESTION FOR CLASSROOM ACTIVITIES

- Before class, have students access information about electronic fetal monitoring from the March of Dimes website. Use this search as a basis for discussion of nursing implications of a systematic approach to fetal monitoring.

SUGGESTION FOR CLINICAL ACTIVITIES

- During the labor and delivery rotation, ask students to do a manual palpation of contraction and a Doppler auscultation of the fetal heart rate with continuous fetal monitoring. Ask them to compare the assessment data obtained.

LEARNING OUTCOME 7

Compare nonreassuring fetal heart rate patterns to appropriate nursing responses.

Concepts for Lecture

1. Nonreassuring fetal heart rate patterns include severe variable decelerations, late decelerations of any magnitude, absence of variability, and prolonged deceleration.
2. Appropriate nursing responses include: notify the physician; administer maternal oxygen; turn mother to the left side; discontinue oxytocin if being administered; monitor FHR continuously; provide explanation to the mother and partner.

POWERPOINT SLIDES 79–84

Figure 18–11. Types and characteristics of early, late, and variable decelerations

Table 18–4. Guidelines for management of variable, late, and prolonged deceleration patterns

SUGGESTION FOR CLASSROOM ACTIVITIES

- Assign students to review Table 18-4. Have the class break into small groups to discuss priority setting with each type of deceleration. Allow time to compare results and have the group arrive at a consensus of priority interventions.

SUGGESTION FOR CLINICAL ACTIVITIES

- Provide students the opportunity to role play therapeutic communications with clients who have a nonreassuring fetal heart rate pattern.

LEARNING OUTCOME 8

Explain the family's responses to electronic fetal monitoring in nursing care management.

Concepts for Lecture

1. Explain the use of electronic fetal monitoring (EFM).
2. Look at the mother prior to looking at the monitor.
3. Record pertinent data on the monitor strip.

POWERPOINT SLIDES 85–90

SUGGESTION FOR CLASSROOM ACTIVITIES

- Discuss how technology can prevent invasive procedures but may adversely impact the nurse-client relationship. The nurse "nurses" the machine and not the client. Have students list ways a nurse can develop a therapeutic relationship with the client and family experiencing electronic fetal monitoring.

SUGGESTION FOR CLINICAL ACTIVITIES

- Ask students to develop a list of nursing diagnoses and expected outcomes for families experiencing electronic fetal monitoring.

GENERAL CHAPTER CONSIDERATIONS

1. Have students study and learn key terms listed at beginning of chapter.
2. Have students complete end-of-chapter exercises either in their book or on the MyNursingKit website.
3. Use the Classroom Response Questions provided in PowerPoint to assess students prior to lecture.

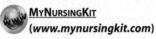

MYNURSINGKIT
(*www.mynursingkit.com*)

- NCLEX RN® review questions
- Case Studies
- Care Plans
- Critical Concept Review
- Thinking Critically
- Weblinks
- Weblink applications
- Nursing Tools
- Audio Glossary
- Images and Tables Library

MYNURSINGLAB
(*www.mynursinglab.com*)

- Knowledge Quick Check
- Pre/Posttests
- Customized study plans
- Images and Tables Library
- *Separate purchase*

CLINICAL SKILLS MANUAL

- *Separate purchase*

PEARSON eTEXT

- Students can search, highlight, take notes, and more all in electronic format
- *Separate purchase*

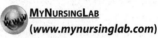

TESTBANK

CHAPTER 19
THE FAMILY IN CHILDBIRTH: NEEDS AND CARE

LEARNING OUTCOME 1

Identify admission data that should be noted when a woman is admitted to the birthing area.

Concepts for Lecture

1. Information obtained during admission is used to develop a clinical pathway for the four stages of labor.
   - Prenatal information.
   - Current assessments.
   - Expected teaching.
   - Nursing care expected for each stage.
   - Expected activity level.
   - Proposed comfort measures.
   - Elimination and nutritional needs.
   - Level of family involvement.

LEARNING OUTCOME 2

Describe the nursing care of a woman and her partner/family upon admission to the birthing area.

Concepts for Lecture

1. The nursing care at admission focuses on providing an orientation to the unit and obtaining an overall physical assessment of the mother that focuses on the well-being of the mother and fetus:
   - Assess the maternal vital signs and FHR.
   - Perform a vaginal exam to determine stage of cervical dilatation and state of membranes.
   - Determine frequency and intensity of contractions.
   - Review systems such as respiratory and neurological.
   - Assess any recent symptoms experienced by the woman.
   - Assess the woman's understanding of the labor process and identification of the woman's support system.

LEARNING OUTCOME 3

Use assessment data to determine the nursing interventions to meet the psychologic, social, physiologic, and spiritual needs of the woman during each stage of labor.

Concepts for Lecture

1. First stage of labor:
   - Establish rapport with the woman and support person.
   - Discuss expectations of labor and delivery.
   - Provide for privacy.
   - Discuss individual expression of pain and discomfort.

 POWERPOINT SLIDES 19–21

 SUGGESTION FOR CLASSROOM ACTIVITIES

- Identify a priority nursing diagnosis and expected outcome for each stage of labor and demonstrate how admission data assists in clinical decision making.

 SUGGESTION FOR CLINICAL ACTIVITIES

- Have students compare the intrapartal clinical pathway with the clinical protocol for a laboring client on their clinical unit.

 POWERPOINT SLIDES 22–26

Table 19–1. Nursing assessments in the first stage

 SUGGESTION FOR CLASSROOM ACTIVITIES

- In many communities, the birthing unit may provide care to non-English-speaking laboring women. Explore the nursing consideration necessary when communication is impacted by language barrier.

 SUGGESTION FOR CLINICAL ACTIVITIES

- Have students complete an admissions assessment on a newly admitted labor client.

 POWERPOINT SLIDES 27–31

Table 19–2. Deviations from normal labor process requiring immediate intervention

 ANIMATION

Placenta Delivery

2. Second stage of labor:
   - Provide as much privacy as possible.
   - Encourage woman and support person to decide who should be present at delivery.
   - Provide praise and encouragement of progress.
3. Third and fourth stages of labor: Refer to Table 19-2.
   - Encourage woman and her support person to hold and look at infant as much as possible.
   - Teach woman the care to be performed after the baby is delivered.
   - Provide the woman with food and fluids as allowed.

VIDEO CLIPS

First Stage of Labor and Transition

VIDEO CLIPS

Second Stage of Labor

VIDEO CLIPS

Third Stage of Labor

VIDEO CLIPS

Fourth Stage of Labor

SUGGESTION FOR CLASSROOM ACTIVITIES

- Discuss how various cultural beliefs may impact nursing assessments during the first stage of labor. Ask student to write a one-page paper reflecting on the incorporation of cultural beliefs their plan of care. Assign "Care Plan: Presence of Extended Family" and "Case Study: Labor and Birth" activities on *mynursingkit.com* as homework.

SUGGESTION FOR CLINICAL ACTIVITIES

- Have students develop a care map for the family of a laboring client. Ask students to include emotional support, comfort measures, supporting breathing techniques, and advocacy. View videos "First Stage of Labor and Transition," "Second Stage of Labor," "Third Stage of Labor," and "Fourth Stage of Labor" on *mynursingkit.com* in class. Have students view animation "Placenta Delivery" on *mynursingkit.com* prior to clinical rotation.

POWERPOINT SLIDES 32–41

Figure 19–2. General comfort

Figure 19–3. Touch as a distraction technique

Table 19–3. Nursing support of patterned-paced breathing

SUGGESTION FOR CLASSROOM ACTIVITIES

- Use "Weblinks: Labor Positions" on *mynursingkit.com* to discuss comfort management during labor.

LEARNING OUTCOME 4

Compare methods of promoting comfort during the first and second stages of labor.

Concepts for Lecture

1. Comfort measures common to the first and second stages of labor include:
   - Client anxiety reduction
   - Client education
   - Relaxation
   - Breathing patterns
   - Instruction for support person
2. Comfort measures specific to the first stage of labor:
   - Pharmacologic agents
   - Epidural
3. Comfort measures specific to the second stage of labor:
   - Effective pushing pattern
   - Rest between pushes

SUGGESTION FOR CLINICAL ACTIVITIES

• Demonstrate breathing techniques. Ask
students to do a return demonstration of
breathing techniques. Ask them what they
see as important points to stress to laboring
clients and their support persons.

LEARNING OUTCOME 5

Explain the immediate needs and physical assessment of the newborn
following birth in the provision of nursing care.

Concepts for Lecture

1. Immediate care of the newborn includes:
   • Respiration
   • Warmth
   • Infection control
   • Identification

POWERPOINT SLIDES 42–46

Figure 19–8. Clearing secretions

Figure 19–9. Umbilical alarm in place
on a newborn infant

Table 19–7. Initial newborn evaluation

VIDEO CLIPS

Newborn Assessment

SUGGESTIONS FOR CLASSROOM ACTIVITIES

• Have a class discussion about the newborn
security measures practiced at clinical sites
in the local community.
• Have students view the video "Newborn
Assessment" on *mynursingkit.com* and refer
to "Skill 5-2: Assigning Newborn Apgar Scores"
in the *Clinical Skills Manual* for review.

SUGGESTION FOR CLINICAL ACTIVITIES

• Incorporate "Skill 5-1: Performing Nasal
Pharyngeal Suctioning" from the *Clinical
Skills Manual* in a clinical conference. Have
students practice this skill on the baby model.

LEARNING OUTCOME 6

Examine the unique needs of the adolescent during birth in the
provision of nursing care.

Concepts for Lecture

1. The adolescent is unique in that she has developmental needs as well
   as physical needs that must be addressed.

POWERPOINT SLIDES 47–49

Figure 19–11. Breastfeeding assistance.
An adolescent mother receives breastfeeding
assistance in the immediate postpartum period

SUGGESTION FOR CLASSROOM ACTIVITIES

• Provide students with a list of community
resources for an adolescent mother. Describe
how these resources can provide assistance to
the adolescent mother.

SUGGESTION FOR CLINICAL ACTIVITIES

• Discuss with students what assessment
information they see as crucial about an
adolescent laboring mother. Assign them to
care for an adolescent mother in labor and
complete a laboring assessment form.

LEARNING OUTCOME 7

Describe the role and responsibilities of the nurse in the management of a precipitous birth.

Concepts for Lecture

1. A precipitous birth is one that occurs rapidly without a physician or certified nurse-midwife in attendance.

GENERAL CHAPTER CONSIDERATIONS

1. Have students study and learn key terms listed at beginning of chapter.
2. Have students complete end-of-chapter exercises either in their book or on the MyNursingKit website.
3. Use the Classroom Response Questions provided in PowerPoint to assess students prior to lecture.

 POWERPOINT SLIDES 50–52

 SUGGESTION FOR CLASSROOM ACTIVITIES

- Describe the emotional needs of the mother who experiences a precipitous birth and how nurses can establish trust and rapport. Discuss what is "ironing the perineum." Discuss infant management during a precipitous birth.

 SUGGESTION FOR CLINICAL ACTIVITIES

- Have students find the emergency birth kit. Ask them to interview a nurse who has delivered a precipitous birth.

 MYNURSINGKIT (*www.mynursingkit.com*)

- NCLEX RN® review questions
- Case Studies
- Care Plans
- Critical Concept Review
- Thinking Critically
- Weblinks
- Weblink applications
- Nursing Tools
- Audio Glossary
- Images and Tables Library

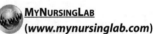 **MYNURSINGLAB** (*www.mynursinglab.com*)

- Knowledge Quick Check
- Pre/Posttests
- Customized study plans
- Images and Tables Library
- *Separate purchase*

CLINICAL SKILLS MANUAL

- *Separate purchase*

 PEARSON eTEXT

- Students can search, highlight, take notes, and more all in electronic format
- *Separate purchase*

 TESTBANK

Chapter 20
Pharmacologic Pain Management

LEARNING OUTCOME 1

Describe the use, administration, dose, onset of action, and adverse effects of systemic drugs to promote pain relief during the nursing care management of the woman in labor and her fetus.

Concepts for Lecture

1. The goal is to provide maximum pain relief with minimum risk to the mother and fetus.
2. After complete assessment, an analgesia agent is generally administered when cervical change has occurred.
3. Drugs may cause fetal respiratory depression at birth if given too late in labor. Additionally, maternal and fetal vital signs must be stable before systemic drugs may be administered. Refer to "Teaching Highlights: What Women Need to Know about Drugs."

LEARNING OUTCOME 2

Compare the major types of regional analgesia and anesthesia, including area affected, advantages, disadvantages, techniques, and nursing care management of the laboring woman and her fetus.

Concepts for Lecture

1. Epidural: Injection of anesthetic agent into the epidural space. Produces little or no feeling to the area from the uterus downward. Pushing during second stage of labor may be impaired due to lack of sensation. Hypotension is the most common side effect. May preload with crystalloid solution bolus. Woman may need urinary catheterization due to the loss of bladder sensation. Assess sensation motor control and orthostatic blood pressure.
2. Continuous epidural analgesia: Provides good analgesia. Produces less nausea and provides a greater ability to cough. May produce breakthrough pain, sedation, and respiratory depression. Itching and hypotension are side effects.
3. Spinal block: A local anesthetic agent is injected directly into the spinal canal. The level of anesthesia is dependent upon level of administration. May be administered higher for the cesarean birth or lower for vaginal birth. The onset of anesthesia is immediate. Side effects include maternal hypotension, which can lead to fetal hypoxia. Requires frequent blood pressure monitoring for health changes. Indwelling urinary catheter is usually needed to decrease bladder sensation and tone. Woman's legs must be protected from injury for 8 to 12 hours after birth of baby due to decreased movement and sensation.

POWERPOINT SLIDES 19–23

Table 20–1. Drug guide: Analgesics used in labor

SUGGESTION FOR CLASSROOM ACTIVITIES

- Have students complete the NCLEX questions on *mynursingkit.com*. Discuss the answers with students at the beginning of the lecture.

SUGGESTION FOR CLINICAL ACTIVITIES

- Have students review clinical protocols on their assigned units related to pain management. Ask them to find a resource on Medlineplus relating to pain management in labor. Ask them to compare and contrast the unit's protocol with the resource from Medlineplus.

POWERPOINT SLIDES 24–36

Figure 20–2. The epidural space lies between the dura mater and the ligamentum flavum, extending from the base of the skull to the end of the sacral canal

Figure 20–3. Technique for lumbar epidural block

Figure 20–5. Pudendal block

Figure 20–6. Local infiltration anesthesia

VIDEO CLIPS

Epidural Placement

SUGGESTION FOR CLASSROOM ACTIVITIES

- Use the video "Epidural Placement" available on *mynursingkit.com* to begin the lecture on regional anesthesia. Start a discussion regarding safety measures required with an epidural placement.

4. Pudendal block: Local anesthesia is injected directly into the pudendal nerve, which produces anesthesia to the lower vagina, vulva, and perineum. Only produces pain relief at the end of labor. Has no effect on the fetus or the progress of labor. May cause hematoma, perforation of the rectum, or trauma to the sciatic nerve.
5. Local infiltration anesthesia: Local anesthesia is injected into the perineum prior to an episiotomy. Provides pain relief only for the episiotomy incision. There is no effect on maternal or fetal vital signs. Requires large amounts of local anesthetic agents.

LEARNING OUTCOME 3

Explain the possible complications of regional anesthesia in nursing care management of the laboring woman and her fetus.

Concepts for Lecture

1. Regional anesthesia administered per spinal or epidural route has similar possible complications: maternal hypotension, bladder distension, inability to push during second stage of labor, severe headache with spinal anesthesia, elevated temperature with epidural anesthesia, possible neurologic damage.

LEARNING OUTCOME 4

Describe the nursing care management for the laboring woman and her fetus related to general anesthesia.

Concepts for Lecture

1. The nurse should assess when the mother ate or drank last, administer prescribed premedication such as an antacid, place a wedge under the mother's right hip to displace the uterus from the vena cava, provide oxygen prior to the start of the surgery, ensure the IV access is established, and assist the anesthesiologist by applying cricoid pressure during the placement of the endotracheal tube.

 SUGGESTION FOR CLINICAL ACTIVITIES

• Examine equipment used during an epidural catheter placement. Demonstrate how the laboring client is positioned.

 POWERPOINT SLIDES 37–39

 SUGGESTION FOR CLASSROOM ACTIVITIES

• Give the students a list of complications of regional anesthesia. Have students develop priority nursing interventions for each complication.

 SUGGESTION FOR CLINICAL ACTIVITIES

• Ask students to develop a teaching plan for a laboring mother and her family regarding complications of regional anesthesia.

 POWERPOINT SLIDES 40–43

Figure 20–7. Cricoid pressure technique. Proper position for fingers in applying cricoid pressure until a cuffed endotracheal tube is placed by the analgesia provider or certified nurse-anesthetist

 SUGGESTION FOR CLASSROOM ACTIVITIES

• Discuss the method of action and side effects of anesthetic agents used in general anesthesia. Emphasize nursing observations and assessments of the laboring mother.

 SUGGESTION FOR CLINICAL ACTIVITIES

• Have students complete drug cards on each of the medications that may be used for "premedication" with general anesthesia. Have students compare the information they obtained on their drug cards to the protocols used on the clinical unit.

LEARNING OUTCOME 5

Describe the major complications of general anesthesia during labor in nursing care management of the woman in labor and her fetus.

Concepts for Lecture

1. Major complications of general anesthesia are fetal depression, uterine relaxation, vomiting, and aspiration.

GENERAL CHAPTER CONSIDERATIONS

1. Have students study and learn key terms listed at beginning of chapter.
2. Have students complete end-of-chapter exercises either in their book or on the MyNursingKit website.
3. Use the Classroom Response Questions provided in PowerPoint to assess students prior to lecture.

 POWERPOINT SLIDES 44–46

 SUGGESTION FOR CLASSROOM ACTIVITIES

- Discuss how the nurse enhances a safe-care environment for the mother who is receiving general anesthesia. Review the "Nursing Practice" boxes in the text and the psychological needs of the mother who has general anesthesia.

 SUGGESTION FOR CLINICAL ACTIVITIES

- Assign students to care for a mother who has just received general anesthesia. Have students develop a problem list in order of priority for a client who has received general anesthesia.

 MYNURSINGKIT
(www.mynursingkit.com)

- NCLEX RN® review questions
- Case Studies
- Care Plans
- Critical Concept Review
- Thinking Critically
- Weblinks
- Weblink applications
- Nursing Tools
- Audio Glossary
- Images and Tables Library

 MYNURSINGLAB
(www.mynursinglab.com)

- Knowledge Quick Check
- Pre/Posttests
- Customized study plans
- Images and Tables Library
- *Separate purchase*

CLINICAL SKILLS MANUAL

- *Separate purchase*

 PEARSON eTEXT

- Students can search, highlight, take notes, and more all in electronic format
- *Separate purchase*

 TESTBANK

CHAPTER 21
CHILDBIRTH AT RISK: PRELABOR COMPLICATIONS

LEARNING OUTCOME 1

Explain the possible causes, risk factors, and clinical therapy for premature rupture of the membranes or preterm labor in determining the nursing care management of the woman and her fetus-newborn.

Concepts for Lecture

1. The exact cause of premature rupture of the membranes (PROM) is unknown. Preterm PROM is associated with infection, multiple pregnancy, bleeding during pregnancy, trauma, and a variety of other factors.
2. PROM nursing care focuses on prevention of infection such as limiting vaginal exams and changing the bed pads frequently.
3. The fetus is monitored carefully.
4. Preterm labor. Nursing care during preterm labor focuses on administration of tocolytics and monitoring for the progression of labor.

LEARNING OUTCOME 2

Compare placenta previa and abruptio placenta, including implications for the mother and fetus, as well as nursing care.

Concepts for Lecture

1. Abruptio placentae is a condition in which the placenta prematurely separates from the uterine wall. It may result in severe hemorrhage; cause death to the mother, the fetus, or both; lead to clotting disorders in the mother. Nursing care involves frequent assessment of uterine tone and measurement of abdominal girth.
2. Placenta previa is a condition in which the placenta implants in the lower segment of the uterus. It may be partially or completely covering the cervical os. Bleeding occurs as the cervix begins to dilate. Bleeding may be mild to severe, depending upon how much of the placenta covers the cervical os. The fetus may develop hypoxia, anemia, or both from the bleeding episode. Nursing care involves assessing blood loss, pain, and uterine contractions. The nurse should never perform a vaginal examination if placenta previa is suspected.

 POWERPOINT SLIDES 20–24

 SUGGESTION FOR CLASSROOM ACTIVITIES

• Assign students to read "Teaching Highlights: Preterm Labor." Ask for student volunteers to role-play a pregnant mother with preterm labor receiving discharge instructions from a student nurse regarding home care.

 SUGGESTION FOR CLINICAL ACTIVITIES

• Review the drug guide on magnesium sulfate with clinical students. Review dosage for preterm labor and related nursing considerations. Bring reflex hammers to clinical. Assign students to demonstrate deep tendon reflexes.

 POWERPOINT SLIDES 25–44

Figure 21–1. Placenta previa

Figure 21–2. Abruptio placentae

Table 21–3. Differential signs and symptoms of placenta previa and abruptio placentae

 SUGGESTION FOR CLASSROOM ACTIVITIES

• Assign students to review Table 21–3. Divide the class into three groups. Assign each group to develop three questions regarding placenta previa and abruptio placenta. Ask each group to allow their classmates to answer their set of questions.

 SUGGESTION FOR CLINICAL ACTIVITIES

• Assign students to care for a client with abruptio placenta/placenta previa in the clinical unit. Ask students to develop a problem list for a neonate of a mother who experienced abruptio placenta/placenta previa.

LEARNING OUTCOME 3

Explain the maternal and fetal-neonatal implications and the clinical therapy in determining the nursing care management of the woman with multiple gestation.

Concepts for Lecture

1. Care of the woman with more than one fetus includes frequent assessment, education of the mother, encouragement of the mother, and preparation of equipment.

LEARNING OUTCOME 4

Compare the identification, maternal and fetal-neonatal implications, clinical therapy, and nursing care management of the woman with hydramnios and oligohydramnios.

Concepts for Lecture

1. Hydramnios: In this condition, the woman has greater than 2000 mL of amniotic fluid. Associated with fetal swallowing and neurologic disorders. Also associated with maternal gestational diabetes, Rh disorders, and multiple gestation pregnancies. Woman may experience shortness of breath and lower extremities edema. Amniocentesis may be performed to remove some of the excessive fluid. The nurse monitors the mother for complications of the amniocentesis and supports the family if fetal disorder is the cause of excess fluid.

2. Oligohydramnios: In this condition, the amount of amniotic fluid is reduced and concentrated. Often found with some renal fetal disorders, fetal postmaturity, and placental insufficiency. May cause fetal respiratory and skeletal abnormalities. May cause prolonged labor. Amnioinfusion may be used during labor to cushion the fetus and umbilical cord. The nurse must continuously monitor the labor pattern for any signs of fetal distress.

 POWERPOINT SLIDES 45–50

Figure 21–3. Twins may be in any of these presentations while in utero

 SUGGESTIONS FOR CLASSROOM ACTIVITIES

- With models, demonstrate various positions of twin gestations in utero. Review Figure 21–3 with students.
- Assign students to complete the NCLEX review questions for this chapter.

 SUGGESTION FOR CLINICAL ACTIVITIES

- Assign students to care for a laboring client who has multiple gestation. Review the intrapartum management of a mother with multiple gestation. Lead a discussion in clinical conference regarding the psychological implications of a multiple gestation pregnancy for a child-bearing family.

 POWERPOINT SLIDES 51–63

 SUGGESTIONS FOR CLASSROOM ACTIVITIES

- Show students sonograms with hydramnios and polydramnios.
- Compare the fetal and neonatal implications of hydramnios and polyhydramnios.

 SUGGESTION FOR CLINICAL ACTIVITIES

- Ask clinical staff to show students the equipment needed for an amnioinfusion. Have students prepare a written care plan for the client with altered amniotic fluid levels.

GENERAL CHAPTER CONSIDERATIONS

1. Have students study and learn key terms listed at beginning of chapter.
2. Have students complete end-of-chapter exercises either in their book or on the MyNursingKit website.
3. Use the Classroom Response Questions provided in PowerPoint to assess students prior to lecture.

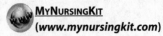

MyNursingKit
(*www.mynursingkit.com*)

- NCLEX RN® review questions
- Case Studies
- Care Plans
- Critical Concept Review
- Thinking Critically
- Weblinks
- Weblinks applications
- Nursing Tools
- Audio Glossary
- Images and Tables Library

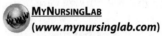

MyNursingLab
(*www.mynursinglab.com*)

- Knowledge Quick Check
- Pre/Posttests
- Customized study plans
- Images and Tables Library
- *Separate purchase*

CLINICAL SKILLS MANUAL

- *Separate purchase*

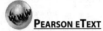

PEARSON eTEXT

- Students can search, highlight, take notes, and more all in electronic format
- *Separate purchase*

TESTBANK

CHAPTER 22
CHILDBIRTH AT RISK: LABOR-RELATED COMPLICATIONS

LEARNING OUTCOME 1

Compare hypertonic and hypotonic labor patterns, including the risks, clinical therapy, and nursing care management.

Concepts for Lecture

1. Hypertonic labor patterns: Characterized by increased frequency and decreased effectiveness of contraction in effacing and dilating the cervix. Usually leads to a prolonged latent phase. May cause the mother to become fatigued and have difficulty coping with the stress of labor. Pattern may cause prolonged pressure on the fetal head. Clinical therapy may involve sedation, pain medication, and bed rest. Pitocin may be given only if CPD and fetal malpresentation are ruled out. Nursing management includes decreasing environmental stimuli, decreasing anxiety, and promoting comfort.

2. Hypotonic labor patterns: Characterized by fewer than 2 to 3 contractions in a 10-minute period during the active phase of labor. The mother may experience fatigue and coping difficulties. The mother is at risk for intrauterine infection and postpartal hemorrhage. Fetus is at risk for sepsis. Clinical therapy includes assessment of adequacy of pelvic measurement and fetal maturity—the use of Pitocin or nipple stimulation once CPD and fetal malpresentation are ruled out. Nursing management includes close monitoring for signs and symptoms of infection and dehydration, and keeping vaginal exams to a minimum.

LEARNING OUTCOME 2

Describe the risks and clinical therapy in determining the nursing care management of postterm pregnancy on the childbearing family.

Concepts for Lecture

1. Postterm pregnancy may result in an increased possibility of labor induction, forceps or vacuum-assisted or cesarean birth, decreased perfusion to the placenta, decreased amount of amniotic fluid and possible cord compression, meconium aspiration, macrosomia or a loss of fat and muscle mass resulting in a small-for-gestational age (SGA) newborn.

POWERPOINT SLIDES 15–41

Figure 22–2. Effects of labor on the fetal head

SUGGESTIONS FOR CLASSROOM ACTIVITIES

- Have students research Active Management of Labor. How does AML differ between Ireland (where it originated) and the U.S. version? Is it a valuable tool? If so, what can nurses do to improve its success here?
- Discuss the role of "therapeutic rest" for prolonged prodromal labor.

SUGGESTIONS FOR CLINICAL ACTIVITIES

- Assign students to care for clients with labor dystocia. Encourage them to actively assist with comfort measures. What helped the most?
- Discuss maternal fatigue and how it related to their clients' contraction patterns.

POWERPOINT SLIDES 42–44

SUGGESTION FOR CLASSROOM ACTIVITIES

- Discuss how a postterm pregnancy impacts a newborn. Discuss the emotional implications of a postterm pregnancy for a mother.

SUGGESTION FOR CLINICAL ACTIVITIES

- Have students review clinical protocols for postterm pregnancy, then develop a plan of care for a mother who has a postterm pregnancy.

LEARNING OUTCOME 3

Relate the various types of fetal malposition and malpresentation to the nursing management for each.

Concepts for Lecture

1. Occiput posterior position: Baby is facing up instead of down as it enters the vagina—may prolong labor. Baby is usually able to be born vaginally but may need forceps assistance to turn the baby.
2. Brow presentation: Forehead of the fetus becomes the presenting part—may cause labor to be prolonged. Cesarean birth necessary if brow presentation persists.
3. Face presentation: Face of the fetus is the presenting part—vaginal birth may be possible, but cesarean birth remains a significant possibility.
4. Breech presentation: Fetal buttock or foot/feet are the presenting part—90% of breech presentations result in cesarean birth.
5. Transverse lie: Fetal shoulder is the presenting part—fetus must be born cesarean.

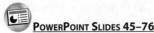
POWERPOINT SLIDES 45–76

Figure 22–3A. Types of cephalic presentations. **A,** The occiput is the presenting part because the head is flexed and the fetal chin is against the chest. The largest anteroposterior (AP) diameter that presents and passes through the pelvis is approximately 9.5 cm

Figure 22–3 B and C. Types of cephalic presentations. **B,** Military presentation. The head is neither flexed nor extended. The presenting AP diameter is approximately 12.5 cm. **C,** Brow presentation. The largest diameter of the fetal head (approximately 13.5 cm) presents in this situation

Figure 22–3D. Types of cephalic presentations. **D,** Face presentation. The AP diameter is 9.5 cm

Figure 22–4. Mechanism of birth in face (mentoanterior) position

Figure 22–5. Face presentation

Figure 22–7. Breech presentation

Figure 22–8. Transverse lie

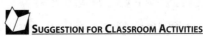
SUGGESTION FOR CLASSROOM ACTIVITIES
- Review your institution's protocols for managing fetal malpresentation. Compare these standards with AWHONN's Standards and Guidelines for Professional Nursing Practice in the Care of Women and Newborns.

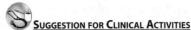
SUGGESTION FOR CLINICAL ACTIVITIES
- Discuss in postconference the care of a laboring client who has a fetal malpresentation. Assign the students a client who has a fetal malpresentation. Have each student develop a priority problem list for this client.

LEARNING OUTCOME 4

Explain the identification, risks, and clinical therapy in determining the nursing care management of the woman and fetus at risk for fetal macrosomia.

Concepts for Lecture

1. Identification of fetal macrosomia is conducted through palpation, ultrasound, and x-ray.
2. Management of fetal macrosomia involves the following: cesarean birth; continuous fetal monitoring; notification of physician, labor dysfunction, or nonreassuring fetal status.

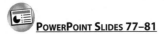
POWERPOINT SLIDES 77–81

SUGGESTION FOR CLASSROOM ACTIVITIES
- Discuss when macrosomia will occur with a pregnancy. Describe the possible complications of labor and birth with macrosomia.

3. Care of the newborn with macrosomia requires assessment.
4. Care of the mother after the birth of a newborn with macrosomia requires fundal massage and close monitoring of vital signs.

LEARNING OUTCOME 5

Relate the maternal implications, clinical therapy, prenatal history, and conditions that may be associated with nonreassuring fetal status to the nursing care of the mother and fetus.

Concepts for Lecture

1. Nursing actions for nonreassuring fetal status include turning the woman, beginning or increasing the IV flow rate, vaginal exam, knee-chest position, discontinuing Pitocin or administering a tocolytic agent, administering oxygen, notifying physician, and obtaining additional information.

LEARNING OUTCOME 6

Describe the nursing care for the mother and fetus with a prolapsed umbilical cord.

Concepts for Lecture

1. Prolapse umbilical cord: Umbilical cord precedes fetal presenting part.
2. Succenturiate placenta: One or more accessory lobes of fetal villi will develop on the placenta.
3. Circumvallate placenta: A double fold of chorion and amnion form a ring around the umbilical cord on the fetal side of the placenta.
4. Battledore placenta: The umbilical cord is inserted at or near the placental margin.
5. Velamentous insertion of the umbilical cord: The vessels of the umbilical cord divide some distance from the placenta in the placental membranes.

 SUGGESTION FOR CLINICAL ACTIVITIES

• Ask students to review health promotion activities for a mother who has had an infant with macrosomia.

 POWERPOINT SLIDES 82–86

Figure 22–9. Intrapartum management of nonreassuring fetal status

 SUGGESTION FOR CLASSROOM ACTIVITIES

• Have students complete exercise in "Thinking Critically: Fetal Heart Rate Tracing." Discuss answers in class. Show examples of nonreassuring tracings.

 SUGGESTION FOR CLINICAL ACTIVITIES

• Show the equipment needed for fetal scalp blood sampling. Demonstrate on a model the acoustic stimulator. Discuss indications and the nursing implications.

 POWERPOINT SLIDES 87–90

Figure 22–11. Knee-chest position is used to relieve cord compression during cord prolapse emergency

 SUGGESTION FOR CLASSROOM ACTIVITIES

• Incorporate the nursing care plan for a client with hemorrhage. Discuss how hemorrhage becomes a concern with each placental and umbilical cord variation.

 SUGGESTION FOR CLINICAL ACTIVITIES

• Show fetal heart tracings of client who experienced prolapsed cord. Have students review "Skill 3-9: Care of the Woman with a Prolapsed Cord" in the *Clinical Skills Manual* prior to clinical. Assign "Care Plan: Prevention of Cord Prolapse" on *mynursingkit.com* for homework.

LEARNING OUTCOME 7

Summarize the identification, maternal and fetal-neonatal implications, clinical therapy, and nursing care management of women with amniotic fluid embolism.

Concepts for Lecture

1. Amniotic fluid embolism: Caused by a small tear in the chorion or amnion high in the uterus, which may allow amniotic fluid to enter the maternal circulatory system. Usually occurs during or after birth. The woman experiences sudden symptoms of respiratory distress leading to severe hemorrhage. This disorder is life threatening.
2. Hydramnios: In this condition, the woman has greater than 2000 mL of amniotic fluid. Associated with fetal swallowing and neurologic disorders. Also, associated with maternal gestational diabetes, Rh disorders, and multiple gestation pregnancies. Woman may experience shortness of breath and lower extremities edema. Amniocentesis may be performed to remove some of the excessive fluid. The nurse monitors the mother for complications of the amniocentesis and supports the family if fetal disorder is the cause of excess fluid.
3. Oligohydramnios: In this condition, the amount of amniotic fluid is reduced and concentrated. Often found with some renal fetal disorders, fetal postmaturity, and placental insufficiency. May cause fetal respiratory and skeletal abnormalities. May cause prolonged labor. Amnioinfusion may be used during labor to cushion the fetus and umbilical cord. The nurse must continuously monitor the labor pattern for any signs of fetal distress.

LEARNING OUTCOME 8

Explain the types, maternal and fetal-neonatal implications, and clinical therapy in determining the nursing care management of the woman with cephalopelvic disproportion.

Concepts for Lecture

1. Labor is usually prolonged in the presence of CPD. Vaginal birth may be possible depending upon the type of CPD. The woman may increase pelvic diameter during labor by squatting, sitting, rolling from side to side, or maintaining a knee-chest position. CPD may make cesarean the only available method of birth.

POWERPOINT SLIDES 91–94

SUGGESTIONS FOR CLASSROOM ACTIVITIES

- Show students sonograms with hydramnios and polydramnios.
- Discuss maternal mortality in the context of current societal values relating to responsibility and blame in obstetrical care. What are realistic outcomes? Who should "pay" if a woman or fetus dies from amniotic embolism? What is the nurse's role in educating the public about realistic expectations for childbirth outcomes?

SUGGESTION FOR CLINICAL ACTIVITIES

- Ask clinical staff to show students the equipment needed for an amnioinfusion. Have students prepare a written care plan for the client with altered amniotic fluid levels.

POWERPOINT SLIDES 95–98

SUGGESTIONS FOR CLASSROOM ACTIVITIES

- Review fetal assessments (Chapter 18) that may be used to assess the presentation and position of the fetus when CPD is suspected.
- Have students list terminology used to describe slow labor and a small pelvis. Explore the subtext of these words and their meaning to a laboring woman. What is the nurse's role in maintaining the couple's confidence in the normalcy of childbirth?

SUGGESTIONS FOR CLINICAL ACTIVITIES

- Invite an experienced labor nurse to speak about the various positions that may be used to increase pelvic diameters in CPD.
- Have students work with laboring clients to optimize pelvic diameter. Compare labors in semi-Fowler's or lithotomy to upright positions.

LEARNING OUTCOME 9

Identify common complications of the third and fourth stages of labor.

Concepts for Lecture

1. The most common complications of the third and fourth stages of labor are retained placenta—if not expelled, the placenta must be manually removed from the uterus; lacerations—suspect when there is bright-red bleeding in the presence of a contracted uterus, usually repaired immediately after the birth of the child; placenta accreta—in this condition, the chorionic villi attach directly to the myometrium of the uterus and may result in maternal hemorrhage and failure of the placenta to separate from the uterus (may result in the need for hysterectomy at time of birth).

POWERPOINT SLIDES 99–110

SUGGESTION FOR CLINICAL ACTIVITIES

- Have students develop a problem list (nursing diagnoses) in order of priority for common complications in the third and fourth stages of labor. Ask the clinical group to develop an expected outcome for each problem/nursing diagnosis.

LEARNING OUTCOME 10

Explain the etiology, diagnosis, and phases of grief in determining the nursing care management of the family experiencing perinatal loss.

Concepts for Lecture

1. Perinatal loss results from three factors: fetal factors, maternal factors, or placental or other factors.
2. Diagnosis may be made by the mother or by the physician.
3. Nursing care involves supporting the family through the grief work.

POWERPOINT SLIDES 111–118

Table 22–2. Tests to determine cause of fetal loss

SUGGESTION FOR CLASSROOM ACTIVITIES

- Bring remembrances kits to class. Discuss the significance to each aspect of the kit. Discuss resources available through the March of Dimes.

SUGGESTION FOR CLINICAL ACTIVITIES

- Have students assist with postmortem care and assessment of a stillborn infant in the nursery. Point out ways in which the infant's dignity is maintained. Acknowledge the staff and student's feelings. Remain with the student and model behavior that supports the nurse's grieving. Discuss the importance of working through grief as nurses. Allow the students to vent their feelings at an appropriate time.

LEARNING OUTCOME 11

Explain the psychologic factors that may contribute to complications during labor and birth in determining the nursing care management.

Concepts for Lecture

1. Psychologic disorders such as depression and acute anxiety may have a profound effect on labor, particularly when complications occur that might jeopardize the mother or fetus.

POWERPOINT SLIDES 66–69

SUGGESTIONS FOR CLASSROOM ACTIVITIES

- Review the coping techniques discussed in Chapter 8. Give examples of nontherapeutic communication during the laboring process. Ask students to react to the nontherapeutic communication.
- Have students list the expected emotional changes and behaviors of pregnancy and compare to the behaviors of women with psychologic disorders. How are they similar and what makes them different?

SUGGESTIONS FOR CLINICAL ACTIVITIES

- Have students develop teaching plans for the nursing diagnosis: Ineffective individual coping related to increased anxiety and stress during the laboring process.
- Review and have students practice therapeutic communication and touch techniques prior to interacting with clients.

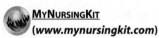 **MYNURSINGKIT**
(*www.mynursingkit.com*)

- NCLEX RN® review questions
- Case Studies
- Care Plans
- Critical Concept Review
- Thinking Critically
- Weblinks
- Weblink applications
- Nursing Tools
- Audio Glossary
- Images and Tables Library

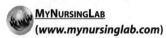 **MYNURSINGLAB**
(*www.mynursinglab.com*)

- Knowledge Quick Check
- Pre/Posttests
- Customized study plans
- Images and Tables Library
- *Separate purchase*

CLINICAL SKILLS MANUAL

- *Separate purchase*

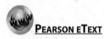 **PEARSON eTEXT**

- Students can search, highlight, take notes, and more all in electronic format
- *Separate purchase*

 TESTBANK

GENERAL CHAPTER CONSIDERATIONS

1. Have students study and learn key terms listed at beginning of chapter.
2. Have students complete end-of-chapter exercises either in their book or on the MyNursingKit website.
3. Use the Classroom Response Questions provided in PowerPoint to assess students prior to lecture.

Chapter 23
Birth-Related Procedures

Learning Outcome 1

Explain the methods, purpose, and contraindications of external and podalic versions that determine nursing care management.

Concepts for Lecture

1. An external version (cephalic version) may be done after 36 weeks' gestation to change a breech presentation to a cephalic presentation: Physician applies external manipulation to the maternal abdomen; fetal part must not be engaged; NST performed to establish fetal well-being.
2. Internal version (podalic version) is used less frequently to turn a second twin during a vaginal birth. It is used only if second fetus does not descend readily and heartbeat is not assuring.

 PowerPoint Slides 20–24

 Suggestion for Classroom Activities

- Assign students to read the "Critical Thinking in Action" section at the end of the chapter and answer the questions there.

 Suggestion for Clinical Activities

- Have students develop a written care plan for the client undergoing version.

Learning Outcome 2

Describe the use of amniotomy and the nursing care management of woman and fetus.

Concepts for Lecture

1. There are several reasons an amniotomy (artificial rupture of the amniotic membranes) is used: To induce labor; to accelerate labor; to apply an internal fetal monitor or insert an intrauterine catheter; or when risks include a prolapsed cord and infection.

 PowerPoint Slides 25–26

 Suggestion for Classroom Activities

- Describe client teaching before an amniotomy as well as priority nursing documentation after an amniotomy.

 Suggestion for Clinical Activities

- Show students an amnihook. Have them review the protocol for amniotomy on their client unit. Discuss nursing observations during the procedure with the group.

Learning Outcome 3

Compare the methods for inducing labor, explaining their advantages and disadvantages in determining the nursing management for women during labor induction.

Concepts for Lecture

1. Cervical ripening may hasten the beginning of labor or shorten the course of labor. It may cause hyperstimulation of the uterus.
2. Stripping the membranes may not induce labor—if labor is initiated, it typically begins within 48 hours—and may cause bleeding.
3. Pitocin infusion is usually effective at producing contractions. It may cause hyperstimulation of uterus.

 PowerPoint Slides 27–33

 Suggestion for Classroom Activities

- Prior to class, assign students to do the "Care Plan" activity on *mynursingkit.com*. Ask them to use the protocol on their assigned unit regarding Pitocin and labor induction as a resource. Discuss answers with class and ask them to compare the unit's protocol with the nursing care plan. Review "Skill 3-7: Assisting with and Monitoring the Woman Undergoing Labor Induction with Pitocin and Cervical Ripening Agents" in the *Clinical Skills Manual*.

SUGGESTION FOR CLINICAL ACTIVITIES

- Before clinical, ask the students to complete the "Thinking Critically: Determining Infusion Rate" exercise. In clinical conference, discuss the answers with the students. Ask them to list three to five key nursing assessments and observations when a client has a Pitocin infusion. Review the Clinical Pathway for induction of labor with clinical students.

 POWERPOINT SLIDES 34–39

Figure 23–2. The two most common types of episiotomies are midline and mediolateral

LEARNING OUTCOME 4

Describe the measures to prevent episiotomy, and the types of episiotomy and associated nursing care management.

Concepts for Lecture

1. Two types of episiotomy are used: midline and mediolateral.
2. During the episiotomy the nurse supports the woman, explaining the procedure. After delivery nursing care: Place an ice pack to the perineum; inspect the perineum frequently; instruct the woman in perineal hygiene, self-care, and comfort measures.

 SUGGESTION FOR CLASSROOM ACTIVITIES

- Review Figure 23-2 with students. Discuss indications for an episiotomy. Review methods to prevent an episiotomy. Have students practice "push, take a breath, push, take a breath," which eases the infant out slowly.

 SUGGESTION FOR CLINICAL ACTIVITIES

- Ask students to prepare a client handout on care after an episiotomy. Discuss handouts in clinical conference. Ask students to present this information to a postpartum client.

 POWERPOINT SLIDES 40–47

Figure 23–3. Application of forceps in occiput anterior (OA) position

LEARNING OUTCOME 5

Explain the indications, maternal, and neonatal risks that impact nursing care management during forceps-assisted birth.

Concepts for Lecture

1. Indications: Shorten the second stage of labor; assist the woman's pushing effort; help with maternal exhaustion, or when regional anesthesia impairs the woman's ability to push effectively.
2. Risks: Newborn bruising, edema, facial lacerations, cephalhematoma, and transient facial paralysis; woman may experience vaginal lacerations, increased bleeding, bruising, and edema.

 SUGGESTION FOR CLASSROOM ACTIVITIES

- Assign student to research guidelines for the use of forceps on the American Academy of Pediatrics and or the American College of Obstetricians and Gynecologists websites prior to class. Ask them to discuss what they have learned about the risks to the mother and fetus.

 SUGGESTION FOR CLINICAL ACTIVITIES

- Show clinical students an outlet forceps, low forceps, and midforceps. Discuss the indication for each type of forceps.

LEARNING OUTCOME 6

Discuss the use of and risk of vacuum extraction use to assist birth.

Concepts for Lecture

1. The vacuum extractor assists birth by applying suction to the fetal head—but may cause cephalhematoma and increases risk for jaundice.

LEARNING OUTCOME 7

Explain the indications for cesarean birth, impact on the family unit, preparation and teaching needs, and associated nursing care.

Concepts for Lecture

1. Most common indications for cesarean birth are fetal distress, lack of labor progression, maternal infection, pelvic size disproportion, placenta previa, and previous cesarean section. Couples should be encouraged to participate in as many choices as possible concerning the surgical birth.
2. Preparation for cesarean birth requires establishing IV lines, placing an indwelling catheter, and performing an abdominal prep.
3. Teaching needs include: What to expect before, during, and after delivery; role of significant others; and interaction with the newborn.
4. Associated nursing care: Routine postpartal care including fundal checks, care of incision, monitoring Intake & Output, assessment of the respiratory system, and assessment of bowel sounds.

POWERPOINT SLIDES 48–50

Figure 23–4A. Vacuum extractor traction. *A,* The cup is placed on the fetal occiput and suction is created. Traction is applied in a downward and outward direction

VIDEO CLIPS

Vacuum Extraction

SUGGESTION FOR CLASSROOM ACTIVITIES

- Show the video "Vacuum Extraction" on *mynursingkit.com* in class. Discuss maternal and fetal risks. If possible, show students a vacuum extractor and a vacuum extractor with a low-profile cup.

SUGGESTION FOR CLINICAL ACTIVITIES

- Assign students to check the FDA website to read the public health advisory on the need for caution in vacuum-assisted deliveries. Ask them to discuss the precautions recommended by the FDA.

POWERPOINT SLIDES 51–59

Figure 23–5. Uterine incisions for a cesarean birth

VIDEO CLIPS

Cesarean Birth

SUGGESTION FOR CLASSROOM ACTIVITIES

- Show the "Cesarean Birth" video on *mynursingkit.com* in class. Discuss indications for a cesarean section. Ask students to discuss key preoperative preparation.

SUGGESTION FOR CLINICAL ACTIVITIES

- Assign students to observe a cesarean birth. Ask clinical students to discuss how nursing promotes the safety of the client before, during, and after the procedure.

LEARNING OUTCOME 8

Examine the risks, guidelines, and nursing care of the woman undergoing vaginal birth following cesarean birth.

Concepts for Lecture

1. Most common risks are: hemorrhage, uterine rupture, infant death.
2. Nursing care: continuous EFM, internal monitoring, and IV fluid. Pitocin induction should be avoided if possible.

GENERAL CHAPTER CONSIDERATIONS

1. Have students study and learn key terms listed at beginning of chapter.
2. Have students complete end-of-chapter exercises either in their book or on the MyNursingKit website.
3. Use the Classroom Response Questions provided in PowerPoint to assess students prior to lecture.

POWERPOINT SLIDES 60–63

SUGGESTION FOR CLASSROOM ACTIVITIES

- Assign students a library assignment to research "A Trial of Labor after a Cesarean Section" and "Vaginal Birth after Cesarean Section." Lead a discussion on the criteria that the mother should meet to reduce complications

SUGGESTION FOR CLINICAL ACTIVITIES

- Assign students to review their assigned clinical facilities guidelines or protocol regarding a "Trial of Labor after a Cesarean Section" and "Vaginal Birth after Cesarean Section."

MYNURSINGKIT
(www.mynursingkit.com)

- NCLEX RN® review questions
- Case Studies
- Care Plans
- Critical Concept Review
- Thinking Critically
- Weblinks
- Weblink applications
- Nursing Tools
- Audio Glossary
- Images and Tables Library

MYNURSINGLAB
(www.mynursinglab.com)

- Knowledge Quick Check
- Pre/Posttests
- Customized study plans
- Images and Tables Library
- *Separate purchase*

CLINICAL SKILLS MANUAL

- *Separate purchase*

PEARSON eTEXT

- Students can search, highlight, take notes, and more all in electronic format
- *Separate purchase*

TESTBANK

CHAPTER 24
THE PHYSIOLOGIC RESPONSES OF THE NEWBORN TO BIRTH

LEARNING OUTCOME 1

Explain the respiratory and cardiovascular changes that occur during the newborn's transition to extrauterine life and during stabilization in determining the nursing care of the newborn.

Concepts for Lecture

1. Newborn respiration is initiated primarily by chemical and mechanical events associated with thermal and sensory stimulation.
2. Onset of respiration stimulates cardiovascular changes. Air enters the lungs, oxygen content rises in alveoli and stimulates relaxation of pulmonary arteries. This leads to decreased vascular resistance that allows complete vascular flow to the lungs.

 POWERPOINT SLIDES 20–30

Figures 24–1. Initiation of respiration in the newborn

Figures 24–2. Transitional circulation

 SUGGESTIONS FOR CLASSROOM ACTIVITIES

- Compare and contrast use of bulb syringe and mucus trap suction during birth.
- List the complications that occur before or during labor and birth which impact lung expansion

 SUGGESTION FOR CLINICAL ACTIVITIES

- Have students compare their newborn's heart and respiratory rate to normal ranges in the text.

LEARNING OUTCOME 2

Compare the factors that modify the newborn's blood values to the corresponding results.

Concepts for Lecture

1. Newborn blood values are affected by the site of the blood sample, gestational age, prenatal and/or perinatal hemorrhage, and timing of the clamping of the umbilical cord.

 POWERPOINT SLIDES 31–36

Table 24–2. Normal term newborn cord blood values

 SUGGESTION FOR CLASSROOM ACTIVITIES

- Compare and contrast the methods to collect venous and capillary samples in the newborn

 SUGGESTION FOR CLINICAL ACTIVITIES

- During the clinical day, review the laboratory results of several newborns with the clinical group. Have students discuss normal and abnormal results and the related nursing implications.

LEARNING OUTCOME 3

Relate the process of thermogenesis in the newborn and the major mechanisms of heat loss to the challenge of maintaining newborn thermal stability.

 POWERPOINT SLIDES 37–41

Figure 24–5. Methods of heat loss

Concepts for Lecture

1. Thermogenesis is achieved by: Increased basal metabolic rate, muscular activity, nonshivering thermogenesis, metabolizing of brown adipose fat.
2. Heat loss is created by: Evaporation (infant is wet from amniotic fluid and/or bath, convection, radiation, conduction).

LEARNING OUTCOME 4

Explain the steps involved in conjugation and excretion of bilirubin in the newborn.

Concepts for Lecture

1. Unconjugated bilirubin: A byproduct of the destruction of red blood cells. Bilirubin is bound to albumin. It is transferred into liver cells and bound to intracellular proteins. These proteins determine the amount of bilirubin uptake into the liver.
2. UDGPT causes unconjugated bilirubin to be attached to glucuronic acid, which produces conjugated bilirubin. This is excreted into the bile ducts, then into the common duct, and finally into the duodenum.
3. Bacteria transforms conjugated bilirubin into urobilinogen in the intestines and stercobilinogen, and it is excreted from the intestinal tract.

LEARNING OUTCOME 5

Identify the reasons a newborn may develop jaundice and nursing interventions to decrease the probability of jaundice.

Concepts for Lecture

Newborns may develop jaundice because of accelerated destruction of fetal RBCs, impaired conjugation of bilirubin, or increased bilirubin reabsorption from the intestinal tract.

SUGGESTION FOR CLASSROOM ACTIVITIES

- Have students review the Evidence-Based Nursing feature and answer the following question: What methods can be used to protect newborns from high decibel levels?

SUGGESTION FOR CLINICAL ACTIVITIES

- Have students develop a nursing care map for a baby using a radiant warmer.

POWERPOINT SLIDES 42–46

Figure 24–7. Conjugation of bilirubin in newborns

SUGGESTION FOR CLASSROOM ACTIVITIES

- Using textbook Figure 24–7 as a basis for discussion, discuss conjugation of bilirubin and how it impacts body systems. Ask the class how this process may differ in the preterm and term infant.

SUGGESTION FOR CLINICAL ACTIVITIES

- Have students check bilirubin levels on assigned babies in the nursery. Discuss normal and high bilirubin levels. Have students discuss what nursing procedures may assist in decreasing the probability of high bilirubin levels.

POWERPOINT SLIDES 47–51

SUGGESTION FOR CLASSROOM ACTIVITIES

- Have students list nursing diagnoses in order of priority for a baby with physiological jaundice. Compare and contrast how jaundice impacts a preterm and term infant.

SUGGESTION FOR CLINICAL ACTIVITIES

- Ask students to develop a teaching plan for a breastfeeding mother related to physiological jaundice that addresses breastfeeding and breast milk jaundice

LEARNING OUTCOME 6

Delineate the functional abilities of the newborn's gastrointestinal tract and liver.

Concepts for Lecture

1. At birth the newborn can digest most simple carbohydrates, proteins, and fats. The newborn has trouble digesting starches.
2. Meconium is passed within 24 to 48 hours after birth and then the newborn begins to have normal bowel movements.
3. The newborn liver is slightly less active than the adult liver. This indicates the liver has a decreased ability to conjugate all of the bilirubin produced by the destruction of fetal RBCs. The liver plays a crucial role in iron storage, carbohydrate metabolism, and coagulation.

LEARNING OUTCOME 7

Relate the development of the newborn's kidneys to the newborn's ability to maintain fluid and electrolyte balance.

Concepts for Lecture

1. The following characteristics of a newborn's kidneys cause difficulty in maintaining fluid and electrolyte balance: Decreased rate of glomerular flow and limited excretion of solutes; limited tubular reabsorptions, limited ability to concentrate urine.
2. Most newborns void within 48 hours of birth.

LEARNING OUTCOME 8

Describe the immunologic response available to the newborn.

Concepts for Lecture

1. The newborn is unable to recognize, localize, and destroy bacteria.
2. The newborn has passive acquired immunity from the mother, which lasts from 4 weeks to 8 months.
3. The newborn begins to produce its own immunity at about 4 weeks of age.

POWERPOINT SLIDES 52–56

Figure 24–9. Newborn stool samples

SUGGESTION FOR CLASSROOM ACTIVITIES

- Discuss typical characteristics of the newborn GI tract. Ask the class to break into small groups and discuss nursing assessments related to the GI tract. Compare group results and have the class prioritize the assessments.

SUGGESTION FOR CLINICAL ACTIVITIES

- Have students check the different types of formula available in the nursery. Have them compare and contrast content of formulas. Ask them to research the different indications for these formulas and report results of the search.

POWERPOINT SLIDES 57–60

Table 24–5. Newborn urinalysis values

SUGGESTION FOR CLASSROOM ACTIVITIES

- Discuss nursing observations needed when the newborn has not voided within 48 hours. Ask students to discuss how they know if the newborn's fluid intake is adequate. What are indicators of bladder distention?

SUGGESTION FOR CLINICAL ACTIVITIES

- Have students observe the urinary function of the newborn. Ask them to document the color and odor of urine and the appearance of the diaper. Ask students to compare observations in clinical conference.

POWERPOINT SLIDES 61–64

SUGGESTION FOR CLASSROOM ACTIVITIES

- Signs and symptoms of infections are subtle in the newborn. With the class, develop a nursing care plan with the diagnoses of high-risk for infection. Brainstorm with the group regarding nursing assessments and interventions.

LEARNING OUTCOME 9

Explain the physiologic and behavioral characteristics of newborn neurologic function, patterns of behavior during the periods of reactivity, and possible nursing interventions.

Concepts for Lecture

1. The first period of reactivity lasts 30 minutes after birth: The newborn is awake and active, appears hungry, has a strong suck; can initiate breastfeeding; vital signs are elevated. The period of inactivity to sleep lasts 30 minutes to 4 hours: The newborn is difficult to awaken; vital signs return to normal. The second period of reactivity lasts 4 to 6 hours after birth: Vital signs are variable; meconium stool is passed; newborn shows a readiness to feed.
2. The behavioral states of the newborn can be divided into the sleep state and the alert state.

LEARNING OUTCOME 10

Describe the normal sensory-perceptual abilities and behavioral states seen in the newborn period and the associated nursing care.

Concepts for Lecture

1. The normal sensory-perceptual abilities of the newborn are: Visual, auditory, olfactory, taste and sucking, and tactile.
2. Some of the behavioral capabilities of the newborn that assist in adaptation to extrauterine life include self-quieting ability and habituation.

SUGGESTION FOR CLINICAL ACTIVITIES

- Ask students to discuss 3 to 5 situations that may place the newborn at risk for infection since the immune system is not fully activated. Ask the group to develop a "consensus" regarding what nurses can teach parents about these situations.

POWERPOINT SLIDES 65–72

Figure 24–10. Mother and newborn gaze at each other

SUGGESTION FOR CLASSROOM ACTIVITIES

- Discuss how periods of reactivity impact newborn feeding.

SUGGESTION FOR CLINICAL ACTIVITIES

- Students should compare periods of reactivity in infants born 12 hours apart. Have the students share their findings in clinical conference.

POWERPOINT SLIDES 73–78

Figure 24–11. Head turning to follow movement

SUGGESTION FOR CLASSROOM ACTIVITIES

- Discuss the importance of doing a newborn hearing screen. Describe what happens if an infant does not pass the hearing screen.

SUGGESTION FOR CLINICAL ACTIVITIES

- Ask students to observe newborns sleeping in the nursery. Ask them to discuss why they think newborns can sleep in a lighted and noisy environment.

GENERAL CHAPTER CONSIDERATIONS

1. Have students study and learn key terms listed at beginning of chapter.
2. Have students complete end-of-chapter exercises either in their book or on the MyNursingKit website.
3. Use the Classroom Response Questions provided in PowerPoint to assess students prior to lecture.

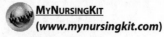

MyNursingKit
(*www.mynursingkit.com*)

- NCLEX RN® review questions
- Case Studies
- Care Plans
- Critical Concept Review
- Thinking Critically
- Weblinks
- Weblink applications
- Nursing Tools
- Audio Glossary
- Images and Tables Library

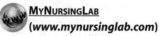

MyNursingLab
(*www.mynursinglab.com*)

- Knowledge Quick Check
- Pre/Posttests
- Customized study plans
- Images and Tables Library
- *Separate purchase*

CLINICAL SKILLS MANUAL

- *Separate purchase*

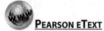

PEARSON eTEXT

- Students can search, highlight, take notes, and more all in electronic format
- *Separate purchase*

TESTBANK

CHAPTER 25
NURSING ASSESSMENT OF THE NEWBORN

LEARNING OUTCOME 1

Describe the physical and neuromuscular maturity characteristics assessed to determine the gestational age of the newborn.

Concepts for Lecture

1. The common physical characteristics included in the gestational age assessment are skin, lanugo, sole (plantar) creases, breast tissues and size, ear form and cartilage, genitalia.
2. The neuromuscular components of gestational age scoring tools are posture, square window sign, popliteal angle, arm recoil, heel-to-toe extension, scarf signs.
3. By assessing the physical and neuromuscular components specified in the gestational age tool, the nurse determines the gestational age of the newborn and identifies the newborn as SGA, AGA, or LGA and prioritizes individual needs.

 POWERPOINT SLIDES 22–40

Figure 25–1. Newborn maturity rating and classification

Figure 25–6. Male genitals

Figure 25–7. Female genitals

Figure 25–8. Square window sign

Figure 25–9. Scarf sign

Figure 25–12. Classification of newborns by birth weight and gestational age

 SUGGESTION FOR CLASSROOM ACTIVITIES

- Review Figure 25-1 with the class. Place emphasis on the square window sign (Figure 25-8) and the scarf sign (Figure 25-9). If possible bring copies of the New Ballard Score and Dubowitz rating scales to class.

 SUGGESTION FOR CLINICAL ACTIVITIES

- Have students complete a gestational age assessment on a newborn. They should compare their results with that of the nursery nurse.

LEARNING OUTCOME 2

Identify the components of a systematic physical assessment of the newborn.

Concepts for Lecture

1. Normal ranges for newborn vital signs include heart rate: 120 to 160 beats per minutes; respiration: 30 to 60 respirations per minute; axillary temperature: 36.1 to 37.2°C (97.5 to 99°F); skin temperature: 36 to 36.5°C (96.8 to 97.7°F); rectal temperature, 36.6 to 37.2°C (97.8 to 99°F); blood pressure at birth: 80-60/45-40 mm Hg.
2. Normal newborn measurements include: Weight range: 2500 to 4000 g (5 lb, 8 oz to 8 lb, 13 oz), with weight dependent on maternal size and age; length range: 46 to 56 cm (18 to 22 in); head circumference range: 32 to 37 cm (12.5 to 14.5 in)—approximately 2 cm larger than the chest circumference.

 POWERPOINT SLIDES 41–74

Figure 25–25. Cephalohematoma

Figure 25–26. Caput succedaneum

Figure 25–34. Umbilical hernia

Figure 25–36. Barlow and Ortolani maneuvers

Table 25–3. Comparison of cephalohematoma and caput succedaneum

Table 25–4. Newborn vital signs

3. The newborn infant should have a head that appears large for its body. The normal newborn has a prominent abdomen, sloping shoulders, narrow hips, and rounded chest. The body appears long and the extremities short.
4. Newborns tend to stay in flexed position and will resist straightening of the extremities. Hands remain clenched. Behaviorally, the infant will sleep the majority of the time and wake for feeding. The infant should be easily consoled when upset.

 SUGGESTION FOR CLASSROOM ACTIVITIES
- Bring several newborn measurements (head, weight, and height) and growth charts to class. Have students practice graphing newborn measurements on the growth charts.

 SUGGESTION FOR CLINICAL ACTIVITIES
- Have students take vital signs and measurements on a newborn. Ask them to compare results with Table 25-4.

LEARNING OUTCOME 3

Describe the normal physical characteristics and normal variations of the newborn and compare abnormal findings to possible causes and nursing responses.

Concepts for Lecture

1. Basis for complete newborn assessment includes: Prenatal history, determination of gestational age, physical assessment, behavioral assessment.
2. Components of a complete newborn physical assessment include: vital signs; weight length and head circumference; skin appearance and presence of birthmarks; examination of the head for size, appearance, symmetry, presence and status of fontanelles; hair appearance; condition and symmetry of face, eyes, and ears; appearance and condition of the nose and mouth; appearance of chest and auscultation of lungs and heart; appearance of abdomen and presence of bowel sounds; inspect umbilical stump for two arteries and one vein; appearance of appropriate genitalia; condition and patency of anus; position and condition of extremities, trunk, and spine.
3. The nurse should be knowledgeable about variations that are indicative of normal newborn responses as well as those that indicate a need for further investigation.
4. An important role of the nurse during the physical and behavioral assessments of the newborn is to teach the parents about their newborn and involve them in their baby's care. This involvement facilitates the parents' identification of their newborn's uniqueness and allays their concern.

 POWERPOINT SLIDES 75-83

Figure 25–16. Axillary temperature measurement

Table 25–2. Newborn measurements

 SUGGESTION FOR CLASSROOM ACTIVITIES
- Demonstrate physical assessment on a newborn/infant in class. Show students how they can access growth charts from the CDC website. Give examples of measurements the students can plot on growth charts.

SUGGESTION FOR CLINICAL ACTIVITIES
- Assign students to teach a new mother about the physical characteristics of her new infant. What do parents need to know to better meet their infant's needs? Demonstrate Ortolani's maneuver or Barlow's maneuver on a baby or model.

LEARNING OUTCOME 4

Describe the components of a neurologic assessment, and the neurologic and neuromuscular characteristics of the newborn and the reflexes that may be present at birth.

Concepts for Lecture

1. Neurologic assessment characteristics are state of alertness, resting position, muscle tone, cry, and motor activity.
2. Neuromuscular assessment characteristics are symmetric movements and strength of all extremities, head lag less than 45 degrees, and ability to hold head erect briefly.
3. Normal reflexes are blink, pupillary reflex, Moro, rooting and sucking, palmar grasp, plantar grasp, stepping, Babinski, tonic neck, prone crawl, trunk incurvation.

 POWERPOINT SLIDES 84-92

Figure 25–40. Moro reflexes

Figure 25–42. Stepping reflex

Newborn Reflex Video Series:
- Maternal Newborn Reflexes Introduction
- Babinski and Plantar Reflex
- Gross and Fine Motor Activity
- Moro Reflex
- Palmar grasp
- Rooting
- Social Behavior and Orientation
- Stepping
- Sucking
- Trunk Incurvation or Galant
- Visual and Audible Tracking
- Vocalization

SUGGESTION FOR CLASSROOM ACTIVITIES

- Before class, assign students to search the Web for information on newborn reflexes. Or assign students to watch some of all of the videos in the Newborn Reflex Video Series on *mynursingkit.com*. Demonstrate neurologic assessment on a newborn or "realistic" newborn model. Then, ask students to relate what they read on newborn reflexes with the instructor demonstration.

SUGGESTION FOR CLINICAL ACTIVITIES

- Have students do a neurological assessment on a newborn. Ask them to compare their results with the normal ranges in the book.

POWERPOINT SLIDES 93–97

SUGGESTION FOR CLASSROOM ACTIVITIES

- Discuss how information from the Brazelton Neonatal Behavioral Assessment can individualize teaching plans for parents.

SUGGESTION FOR CLINICAL ACTIVITIES

- Ask students to observe sleep-wake patterns and to see how rapidly the newborn moves from one state to another. Ask students to document if the newborn can be consoled.

POWERPOINT SLIDES 98–100

Figure 25–43. Self-soothing

LEARNING OUTCOME 5

Describe the components of the newborn behavioral assessment and the normal behavioral characteristics and normal variations of the newborn.

Concepts for Lecture

1. The categories of the newborn behavioral assessment are: Habitation, orientation to inanimate and animate visual and auditory assessment stimuli; motor activity; frequency of alert states, state changes, color changes, activity, and peaks of activity, self quieting activity; cuddliness.

LEARNING OUTCOME 6

Correlate findings in newborn behavioral assessment to possible nursing responses and to teach and involve parents in the care of their newborn.

Concepts for Lecture

1. Behaviorally, the infant will sleep the majority of the time and wake for feeding. The infant should be easily consoled when upset.

2. An important role of the nurse during the behavioral assessment is to teach newborn parents about their newborn and involve them in their baby's care. This involvement facilitates the parent's identification of their newborn's uniqueness, allays their concerns, and fosters positive attachment experiences.

GENERAL CHAPTER CONSIDERATIONS

1. Have students study and learn key terms listed at beginning of chapter.
2. Have students complete end-of-chapter exercises either in their book or on the MyNursingKit website.
3. Use the Classroom Response Questions provided in PowerPoint to assess students prior to lecture.

SUGGESTIONS FOR CLASSROOM ACTIVITIES

- Assign students to complete the Critical Thinking in Action case study at the end of the chapter. Discuss answers in class.
- Show class pictures of babies in an alert state. Explain how parents can use the alert state to interact and perform child care activities.

SUGGESTIONS FOR CLINICAL ACTIVITIES

- Assign students to review Figure 25–43. Ask students to develop a teaching plan on a newborn's "self-soothing activities" and to teach the information to their assigned client.
- In clinical conference, lead a discussion on the concept "rooming-in" and how it fosters attachment and bonding.

MYNURSINGKIT (www.mynursingkit.com)

- NCLEX RN® review questions
- Case Studies
- Care Plans
- Critical Concept Review
- Thinking Critically
- Weblinks
- Weblink applications
- Nursing Tools
- Audio Glossary
- Images and Tables Library

MYNURSINGLAB (www.mynursinglab.com)

- Knowledge Quick Check
- Pre/Posttests
- Customized study plans
- Images and Tables Library
- *Separate purchase*

CLINICAL SKILLS MANUAL

- *Separate purchase*

PEARSON ETEXT

- Students can search, highlight, take notes, and more all in electronic format
- *Separate purchase*

TESTBANK

CHAPTER 26
THE NORMAL NEWBORN: NEEDS AND CARE

LEARNING OUTCOME 1

Summarize essential information to be obtained about a newborn's birth experience and immediate postnatal period.

Concepts for Lecture

1. Information is gathered from the following sources on the condition of the newborn: Apgar scores, any resuscitation effort, vital signs, voiding, passage of meconium.
2. Labor and birth record: Length and course of labor, type of delivery, conditions at delivery, medications given during labor.
3. Antepartal record: Infections during pregnancy, estimated date of birth (EDB), previous pregnancies, any congenital anomalies, HIV test result.
4. Parent-newborn interaction information: Type of infant feeding desired, desire for circumcision if infant is male, support system available, whether rooming-in is desired.

LEARNING OUTCOME 2

Explain how the physiologic and behavioral responses of the newborn during the first 4 hours after birth (admission and transitional period) determine the nursing care of the newborn.

Concepts for Lecture

1. Maintenance of a clear airway and stable vital signs: The infant's cardiovascular and respiratory systems are changing rapidly: the infant is dried and stimulated to breathe; free-flow oxygen is available to assist the infant's transition. Apgar score and vital signs are used to assess the infant's transition.
2. Maintenance of a neutral thermal environment: The infant is stressed by the change from the warm, moist environment of the uterus to the dry, drafty environment of the delivery room and nursery; a neutral thermal environment is needed to prevent the need for increased oxygen and calories; the newborn is dried and placed under a radiant warmer; a cap is placed on the infant's head to prevent heat loss; temperature is checked frequently and the infant is kept from drafts and open windows.
3. Prevention of hemorrhagic disease in the newborn: Newborn lacks intestinal bacterial flora, which is necessary for the production of vitamin K; prothrombin levels are low during the first few days of life; vitamin K injection is given IM quickly after birth.
4. Prevention of eye infection: Infant may come in contact with infected material during birth; eye prophylaxis is given to all newborns to prevent serious eye infection.

 POWERPOINT SLIDES 19–24

Table 26–1. Signs of newborn transition

 SUGGESTION FOR CLASSROOM ACTIVITIES

- Discuss the family adjustments that must be made after the birth of a newborn. Describe how parents can enhance infant attachment.

 SUGGESTION FOR CLINICAL ACTIVITIES

- Have students assist with the admission of a newborn to the nursery. Have them develop a priority nursing diagnoses list for the newborn just admitted to the nursery.

 POWERPOINT SLIDES 25–40

Figure 26–2. Temperature monitoring for the newborn

Figure 26–3. Procedure for vitamin K injection

Figure 26–4. Injection sites

Figure 26–5. Ophthalmic ointment

Table 26–1. Signs of newborn transition

Table 26–3. Signs of newborn distress

 VIDEO CLIPS

Newborn Care

 SUGGESTIONS FOR CLASSROOM ACTIVITIES

- Review Apgar Score while discussing Table 26-1. Signs of Newborn Transition.
- Assign students to complete the NCLEX review questions on *mynursingkit.com* to submit to instructor.

5. Assessment of neonatal distress: The nurse assesses and teaches parents signs and symptoms of respiratory distress such as tachypnea, grunting, retractions, or change in color; parents are taught use of the bulb syringe and proper positioning to prevent respiratory problems.
6. Expected periods of reactivity: The infant is usually alert for the first hour after birth; the nurse should encourage eye-to-eye contact between the infant and the parents; nurse should initiate first feedings if infant is stable.

Learning Outcome 3

Describe the major nursing considerations and activities to be carried out after the transitional period until discharge based on the physiologic and behavioral responses of the newborn.

Concepts for Lecture

1. Nursing interventions during the first four hours after birth include: Monitor vital signs; assess and monitor skin color; assess condition of cord; assess weight, length, and head circumference; assess extremity movement; determine gestational age classification; assess for the presence of any anomalies; identify infant and initiate security system; check for expected reflexes; assess ability to suck and swallow; bathe infant when temperature is stable; assist mother to feed as soon as infant is stable; administer necessary medications.
2. Subsequent daily care includes: Monitor vital signs every 6 to 8 hours; assess condition of umbilical cord; initiate hearing screening if applicable; assess infant's ability to void and stool; determine if infant is feeding adequately; swaddle infant to provide for warmth; initiate necessary immunizations; initiate newborn screening tests; provide teaching to parents concerning newborn care.

Learning Outcome 4

Describe common concerns of families and related content to be included in parent teaching on daily newborn and infant care and discharge planning.

Concepts for Lecture

1. Most parents are concerned about the immediate health of the newborn; measures taken to ensure infant safety; how to provide general infant care; how to properly feed infant.
2. Parent teaching of newborn and infant care includes:
   • Safety measures.
   • Voiding and stool characteristics and patterns.
   • Cord care.
   • Male genitalia care.
   • How to awaken infant.
   • How to quiet infant.
   • Signs of illness.

Suggestions for Clinical Activities
• Ask students to review the clinical agency's protocols for newborns at the time of admission to the nursery (e.g., eye prophylaxis, vitamin K injection, and hepatitis immunization).
• Review the administration of eye ointment and the administration of a IM injection to a newborn.

PowerPoint Slides 41–43

Suggestions for Classroom Activities
• Demonstrate how expected reflexes are checked on a newborn using an infant if possible or a model.
• Demonstrate how to measure head circumference, weight, and length of the baby.

Suggestions for Clinical Activities
• Assign students to observe a nurse completing a newborn admission procedure.
• Ask students to share observation in clinical conference.
• Ask students how the nurse maintained a neutral thermal environment during the procedures.

PowerPoint Slides 44–60

Figure 26–6. Routine umbilical cord care

Figure 26–9. Following circumcision, petroleum ointment may be applied to the site for the next few diaper changes

Suggestions for Classroom Activities
• Discuss measures at local healthcare facilities to ensure newborn safety. Delineate how new parents can make a home secure for a newborn.
• Assign two students to role play a nurse teaching a new mother how to quiet an infant.

Suggestion for Clinical Activities
• Ask students to develop a list of community resources for car seats. Have them review the procedure for securing these car seats for parents with a need. Ask students to compare safety, weight, and height ratings for these car seats.

LEARNING OUTCOME 5

Discuss opportunities to individualize parent teaching and enhance each parent's abilities and confidence while providing infant care in the birthing unit.

Concepts for Lecture

1. Individualized parent teaching is best accomplished by observation and demonstration of common infant activities.

GENERAL CHAPTER CONSIDERATIONS

1. Have students study and learn key terms listed at beginning of chapter.
2. Have students complete end-of-chapter exercises either in their book or on the MyNursingKit website.
3. Use the Classroom Response Questions provided in PowerPoint to assess students prior to lecture.

POWERPOINT SLIDES 61–65

Figure 26–11. Parental confidence

Table 26–4. When parents should call their healthcare provider

SUGGESTIONS FOR CLASSROOM ACTIVITIES

- Have students read the Critical Thinking in Action for Chapter 26 and answer the questions that follow.
- Assign students to review Table 26-4: When Parents Should Call Their Healthcare Provider. Ask for two students to volunteer role playing a new father asking questions regarding what temperature constitutes a fever in a new baby.

SUGGESTION FOR CLINICAL ACTIVITIES

- Ask students to review the various teaching handouts on the unit as well as the videos. Ask them to evaluate whether a demonstration by the nursing staff would enhance the videos or teaching handouts.

MYNURSINGKIT
(www.mynursingkit.com)

- NCLEX RN® review questions
- Case Studies
- Care Plans
- Critical Concept Review
- Thinking Critically
- Weblinks
- Weblink applications
- Nursing Tools
- Audio Glossary
- Images and Tables Library

MYNURSINGLAB
(www.mynursinglab.com)

- Knowledge Quick Check
- Pre/Posttests
- Customized study plans
- Images and Tables Library
- *Separate purchase*

CLINICAL SKILLS MANUAL

- *Separate purchase*

PEARSON eTEXT

- Students can search, highlight, take notes, and more all in electronic format
- *Separate purchase*

TESTBANK

CHAPTER 27
NEWBORN NUTRITION

LEARNING OUTCOME 1

Compare the nutritional value and composition of breast milk and formula preparations in relation to the nutritional needs of the newborn.

Concepts for Lecture

1. Composition of breast milk: 10% solids consisting of carbohydrates, proteins, and fats. 90% is water.
2. Breast milk has immunologic and nutritional biodegradable properties that make it the optimal food for the first year of life.
3. Most common cow's milk protein-based formulas attempt to duplicate the same concentration of carbohydrates, proteins, and fats as 20 kcal/oz breast milk.

LEARNING OUTCOME 2

Explain the advantages and disadvantages of breastfeeding and formula-feeding in determining the nursing care of both mother/family and newborn.

Concepts for Lecture

1. Advantages of breastfeeding: Provides immunologic protection; infants digest and absorb components of breast milk easier; provides more vitamins to infant if mother's diet is adequate; strengthens the mother-infant attachment; no additional cost; breast milk requires no preparation.
2. Disadvantages of breastfeeding: Many medications pass through to breast milk; father unable to equally participate in actual feeding of infant; mother may have difficulty being separated from infant.
3. Advantages of formula-feeding: Provides good nutrition to infant; father can participate in infant feeding patterns.
4. Disadvantages of formula-feeding: May need to try different formulas before finding one that is well-tolerated by the infant; proper preparation is necessary for nutritional adequacy.

PowerPoint Slides 21–25

Table 27–3. Storage guidelines for breast milk and formula

SUGGESTION FOR CLASSROOM ACTIVITIES

- Invite a lactation consultant to class to present information on breastfeeding.

SUGGESTION FOR CLINICAL ACTIVITIES

- Have students attend a La Leche meeting or a breastfeeding class. In postconference, let them report their observations regarding the type of information and support offered at the meeting.

PowerPoint Slides 26–31

Figure 27–6. C-hold hand position

Table 27–2. Types of breast pumps and indications for use

SUGGESTIONS FOR CLASSROOM ACTIVITIES

- Bring to class various types of infant formula and bottles. Bring various types of breast pumps and related equipment to class. Discuss the use, advantages, and disadvantages of the different equipment. Reinforce information in Table 27-2.
- Incorporate a list of community resources on nutrition into the lecture. Discuss with students how their clients can benefit from these resources.

SUGGESTION FOR CLINICAL ACTIVITIES

- Have students work with nursery nurses to learn more about resources for bottle-feeding and breastfeeding. Assign students to a WIC clinical. Ask them to document in a journal the different types of teaching that families receive.

LEARNING OUTCOME 3

Develop guidelines for helping both breast- and formula-feeding mothers to feed their newborns successfully in hospital and community-based settings.

Concepts for Lecture

1. The breastfeeding mother needs to know: How breast milk is produced; how to correctly position the infant for feeding; the procedures for feeding the infant; how to express leaking milk; how to express and store breast milk; how and when to supplement with formula; how to care for the breasts; what medications pass through the breast milk; what kind of support groups are available for breastfeeding.
2. The bottle-feeding mother needs to know: Types of formula available and how to prepare each type; the procedure for feeding the infant; how to correctly position the infant for bottle feeding; how to safely store the formula; how to safely care for bottles and nipples.

 POWERPOINT SLIDES 32–42

Figure 27–2. Modified cradle position

Figure 27–3. Cradle position

Figure 27–4. Football hold position

Figure 27–5. Side-lying position

Figure 27–6. C-hold hand position

Figure 27–7. Scissor hold hand position

Figure 27–8. Nose to nipple

Table 27–1. Comparison of breastfeeding and formula feeding

 VIDEO CLIPS

Nursing in Action: Breastfeeding

 SUGGESTIONS FOR CLASSROOM ACTIVITIES

- Have students review "Actions and Effects of Selected Drugs during Breastfeeding" in the Nursing Tools section on *mynursingkit.com*
- Review Table 27–1 and stress the maternal health, psychologic aspects, and cost of breast feeding and bottle feeding.

 SUGGESTION FOR CLINICAL ACTIVITIES

- Have students complete the Critical Thinking scenario. The clinical group should discuss answers to the questions, and as a group develop priority nursing diagnoses for the mother and infant.

LEARNING OUTCOME 4

Explain the influence of cultural values on infant care, especially feeding practices, in nursing care of the newborn, mother, and family.

Concepts for Lecture

1. Nurse must recognize that cultural values influence infant feeding practices. Be sensitive to ethnic backgrounds of minority populations. Understand that the dominant culture in any society defines normal maternal infant feeding.

 POWERPOINT SLIDES 43–44

 SUGGESTION FOR CLASSROOM ACTIVITIES

- Incorporate developing cultural competence in the breastfeeding lecture. Discuss the impact of culture on specific feeding practices. Have students review "Developing Cultural Competencies: Breastfeeding in Other Cultures" in Chapter 27 for homework.

SUGGESTION FOR CLINICAL ACTIVITIES

- Assign students to research different cultures and how they view breastfeeding. Have students report on their research in clinical conference.

LEARNING OUTCOME 5

Explain the nutritional needs and normal growth patterns of infants and educate parents on these topics.

Concepts for Lecture

1. Parents need to know: Amount of formula to feed infant at each feeding and how often to feed infant; number of times per day the breast-fed infant should be put to the breast; the expected weight gain of both formula- and breastfed infants; the proper diet for the breastfeeding mother.

GENERAL CHAPTER CONSIDERATIONS

1. Have students study and learn key terms listed at beginning of chapter.
2. Have students complete end-of-chapter exercises either in their book or on the MyNursingKit website.
3. Use the Classroom Response Questions provided in PowerPoint to assess students prior to lecture.

 POWERPOINT SLIDES 45–47

 SUGGESTIONS FOR CLASSROOM ACTIVITIES

- Show students infant growth charts. Have the students plot height and weight on the charts. Demonstrate different feeding positions for bottle- and breastfeeding.
- Have students examine breastfeeding information and bottle-feeding information. Have them discuss how this information differs and how it is similar.

 SUGGESTION FOR CLINICAL ACTIVITIES

- Assign students to rotate through a WIC clinic to observe nutritional assessment and counseling. After the observational experience, ask students to summarize the nutritional needs of the family with a newborn.

 MYNURSINGKIT (*www.mynursingkit.com*)

- NCLEX RN® review questions
- Case Studies
- Care Plans
- Critical Concept Review
- Thinking Critically
- Weblinks
- Weblink applications
- Nursing Tools
- Audio Glossary
- Images and Tables Library

 MYNURSINGLAB (*www.mynursinglab.com*)

- Knowledge Quick Check
- Pre/Posttests
- Customized study plans
- Images and Tables Library
- *Separate purchase*

CLINICAL SKILLS MANUAL

- *Separate purchase*

 PEARSON ETEXT

- Students can search, highlight, take notes, and more all in electronic format
- *Separate purchase*

 TESTBANK

CHAPTER 28
THE NEWBORN AT RISK: CONDITIONS PRESENT AT BIRTH

LEARNING OUTCOME 1

Explain the factors present at birth that indicate an at-risk newborn.

Concepts for Lecture

1. Maternal low socioeconomic level: Decreased access to health care; exposure to environmental dangers, such as toxic chemicals and illicit drugs. Refer to Figure 28–1 in the text.
2. Preexisting maternal conditions: Heart disease, diabetes, hypertension, renal disease; maternal age and parity.
3. Pregnancy complications: Abruptio placentae; placenta previa; PIH.

LEARNING OUTCOME 2

Compare the underlying etiologies of the physiologic complications of small-for-gestational-age (SGA) newborns and preterm appropriate-for-gestational-age (Pr AGA) newborns and the nursing care management for each.

Concepts for Lecture

1. Many of the same factors contribute to the common complications of the SGA newborn and the Pr AGA newborn: Maternal factors—grand multiparity; multiple gestation pregnancy; low socioeconomic status; poor maternal nutrition.
2. Maternal disease: Heart disease, hypertension, preeclampsia.
3. Environmental factors: Maternal use of drugs, exposure to toxins, high altitude.
4. Placental factors: Small placenta, placenta previa, abnormal cord insertions.
5. Fetal factors: Congenital infections, chromosomal syndromes.

LEARNING OUTCOME 3

Describe the impact of maternal diabetes mellitus on the newborn.

Concepts for Lecture

1. Infants of diabetic mothers (IDMs) are considered at-risk and require close observation the first few hours and days of life. The most common complications of maternal diabetes mellitus are: hypoglycemia; hypocalcemia; hyperbilirubinemia; birth trauma; polycythemia; respiratory distress syndrome; congenital birth defects—cardiac anomalies, gastrointestinal anomalies, sacral agenesis.

POWERPOINT SLIDES 19–22

Figure 28–1. Newborn classification and neonatal mortality risk chart

SUGGESTION FOR CLASSROOM ACTIVITIES
- Demonstrate neonatal classification and neonatal mortality risk chart.

SUGGESTION FOR CLINICAL ACTIVITIES
- Ask students to develop a nursing care plan for the at-risk newborn, which addresses stressful physiologic conditions and how to conserve the at-risk newborn's energy.

POWERPOINT SLIDES 23–28

SUGGESTION FOR CLASSROOM ACTIVITIES
- Develop a list of toxins and drugs that may have adverse effects on a newborn.

SUGGESTION FOR CLINICAL ACTIVITIES
- Have students rotate through a perinatal clinic setting to observe tests that assist in identifying at-risk newborns.

POWERPOINT SLIDES 29–34

Figure 28–4. Macrosomic infant of a class B insulin-dependent diabetic mother born at 38 weeks' gestation weighing 3402 grams

SUGGESTION FOR CLASSROOM ACTIVITIES
- Identify which cultural groups may have a higher incidence of macrosomia.

LEARNING OUTCOME 4

Compare the characteristics and potential complications that influence nursing care management of the postterm newborn and the newborn with postmaturity syndrome.

Concepts for Lecture

1. Postterm newborn: Applies to any newborn born after 42 weeks' gestation; most are of normal size and health; large fetus may have difficult time passing through the birth canal.
2. Postmaturity syndrome, in which the fetus is exposed to poor placental function, impairs nutrition and oxygenation, and has the following characteristics: hypoglycemia; meconium aspiration; polycythemia; congenital anomalies; seizure activity; cold stress.

LEARNING OUTCOME 5

Discuss the physiologic characteristics of the preterm newborn that predispose each body system to various complications and that are used in developing a plan of care that includes nutritional management.

Concepts for Lecture

1. The major problem of the preterm newborn is the variable immaturity of all systems. The degree of immaturity depends on the length of gestation.
2. Respiratory difficulties.
3. Cardiac difficulties.
4. Temperature control difficulties.
5. Gastrointestinal difficulties.
6. Renal difficulties.
7. Reactivity and behavioral state difficulties.

SUGGESTION FOR CLINICAL ACTIVITIES

• Discuss the common complications that the newborn of a diabetic mother will experience. Ask students to develop a list of nursing diagnoses that are a priority for a newborn of a diabetic mother.

POWERPOINT SLIDES 35–39

Figure 28–5. Postterm infant demonstrates deep cracking and peeling of skin

SUGGESTION FOR CLASSROOM ACTIVITIES

• Delineate which procedures may be done on a postmature infant. Discuss crucial elements of an assessment of a postmature infant.

SUGGESTION FOR CLINICAL ACTIVITIES

• Develop a priority nursing diagnoses list for an infant with post maturity syndrome. Ask the students as a group to develop expected outcomes for each nursing diagnosis.

POWERPOINT SLIDES 40–48

Figure 28–10. Father participating in feeding experience with his premature infant

SUGGESTION FOR CLASSROOM ACTIVITIES

• Review the relationship of the L/S ratio and surfactant. Demonstrate on a model of fetal circulation where the patent ductus arteriosus is. Discuss how renal considerations impact drug selection in preterm infants. Describe the developmental care of the preterm infant.

SUGGESTION FOR CLINICAL ACTIVITIES

• Ask a nursery nurse to discuss with students the equipment used to maintain a neutral thermal environment in the nursery. Have students observe reactivity periods of a preterm infant in the nursery.

Learning Outcome 6

Summarize the nursing assessments of and initial interventions for a newborn with selected congenital anomalies.

Concepts for Lecture

1. Nursing assessments and initial interventions focus on: Respiratory.
2. Neurologic. Refer to Table 28–2.
3. Parental involvement.

PowerPoint Slides 49–56

Figure 28–8. Measuring gavage tube length

Figure 28–9. Auscultation for placement of gavage tube

Figure 28–12. Family bonding occurs when parents have opportunities to spend time with their infant

Table 28–2. Congenital anomalies: identification and care in the newborn period

Suggestion for Classroom Activities

- Discuss immediate nursing assessment measures at birth. Discuss the support that the childbearing family needs if their infant has a congenital anomaly.

Suggestion for Clinical Activities

- Allow students to tour a newborn intensive care unit. Show them resources available to family members. Have students review "Skill 15-3: Administering a Gavage Feeding" in the *Clinical Skills Manual*. Show students the equipment needed for a gavage feeding.

Learning Outcome 7

Explain the special care needed by an alcohol- or drug-exposed newborn.

Concepts for Lecture

1. Special care of the infant who was exposed to drugs or alcohol focuses on: Assessment of the mother's last drug intake and dosage; assessment of congenital anomalies and complications; assessment for signs and symptoms of withdrawal. Refer to Table 28–3.

PowerPoint Slides 57–62

Figure 28–14. Nonnutritive sucking on a pacifier has a calming effect on the newborn

Table 28–3. Neonatal abstinence score sheet

Suggestion for Classroom Activities

- Demonstrate how the neonatal abstinence sheet is scored. Using "Nursing Care Plan: Newborn of a Substance-Abusing Mother," discuss priority nursing care for the newborn of a substance-abusing mother. Discuss how fetal alcohol syndrome can be prevented.

Suggestion for Clinical Activities

- Have students present a nursing article that addresses substance abuse in pregnancy and its impact on the newborn. Encourage students to evaluate the implications for nursing care.

LEARNING OUTCOME 8

Correlate the effects of maternal HIV/AIDS on the infant in the neonatal period and the issues for caregivers of infants at risk for HIV/AIDS in determining hospital-based and community-based nursing care management.

Concepts for Lecture

1. Transmission of HIV/AIDS during the perinatal and neonatal periods can occur across the placenta or through breast milk or contaminated blood. Infant of the mother who has HIV/AIDS receives the same care as all newborn infants. The nurse also includes the following aspects of care: Use standard precautions when drawing blood samples; use disposable gloves when changing diapers; protect infant from opportunistic diseases; keep newborn well-nourished to prevent failure to thrive.

LEARNING OUTCOME 9

Identify the physical examination findings during the early newborn period that would make the nurse suspect a congenital cardiac defect or congestive heart failure.

Concepts for Lecture

1. The three most common manifestations of cardiac defects are cyanosis, detectable heart murmur, and signs of congestive heart failure.

 POWERPOINT SLIDES 63–66

 SUGGESTION FOR CLASSROOM ACTIVITIES

- Discuss the opportunistic infections that may impact the newborn of a mother who has HIV/AIDS.

 SUGGESTION FOR CLINICAL ACTIVITIES

- Discuss the nutritional needs of a newborn of a mother who has HIV/AIDS. In clinical conference, ask students how they would discuss these nutritional needs with family members.

 POWERPOINT SLIDES 67–70

 SUGGESTION FOR CLASSROOM ACTIVITIES

- Review the genetic and environmental factors that increase the risk of a congenital heart anomaly.

 SUGGESTION FOR CLINICAL ACTIVITIES

- Have students research Internet resources on congenital heart defects. In clinical conference, ask them to report on the relevance of the congenital heart defect resource.

GENERAL CHAPTER CONSIDERATIONS

1. Have students study and learn key terms listed at beginning of chapter.
2. Have students complete end-of-chapter exercises either in their book or on the MyNursingKit website.
3. Use the Classroom Response Questions provided in PowerPoint to assess students prior to lecture.

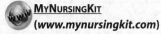

MyNursingKit
(*www.mynursingkit.com*)

- NCLEX RN® review questions
- Case Studies
- Care Plans
- Critical Concept Review
- Thinking Critically
- Weblinks
- Weblink applications
- Nursing Tools
- Audio Glossary
- Images and Tables Library

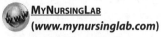

MyNursingLab
(*www.mynursinglab.com*)

- Knowledge Quick Check
- Pre/Posttests
- Customized study plans
- Images and Tables Library
- *Separate purchase*

CLINICAL SKILLS MANUAL

- *Separate purchase*

PEARSON eTEXT

- Students can search, highlight, take notes, and more all in electronic format
- *Separate purchase*

TESTBANK

CHAPTER 29
THE NEWBORN AT RISK: BIRTH-RELATED STRESSORS

LEARNING OUTCOME 1

Discuss how to identify infants in need of resuscitation and the appropriate method of resuscitation based on the labor record and observable physiologic indicators.

Concepts for Lecture

1. Infants at risk for resuscitation include: Nonreassuring fetal heart pattern, meconium-stained amniotic fluid and/or acidosis detected by fetal scalp sample; cardiac disease diagnosed prenatally; other congenital abnormality diagnosed prenatally; premature birth; infant of multiple pregnancy; prolonged or difficult delivery.
2. Infants at need for resuscitation: Weak cry at birth; poor respiratory effort at birth; retractions at birth.
3. Resuscitation methods: Stimulation by rubbing the newborn's back; use of positive pressure to inflate the lungs; endotracheal intubation; medications: Nalaxone (Narcan) may be used to reverse effects of narcotics given to mother prior to birth.

POWERPOINT SLIDES 19–27

Figure 29–1. Demonstration of resuscitation of a newborn with bag and mask

Figure 29–2. External cardiac massage

SUGGESTION FOR CLASSROOM ACTIVITIES

• Discuss the various procedures that may be done as part of the resuscitation of a newborn. Discuss with the students the nursing implications with each procedure.

SUGGESTION FOR CLINICAL ACTIVITIES

• Have the clinical group locate and evaluate emergency equipment on the obstetric unit. Ask students to research and discuss neonatal advanced life support and have them correlate aspects of neonatal advanced life support with the equipment they have located.

LEARNING OUTCOME 2

Based on clinical manifestations, differentiate among the various types of respiratory distress (respiratory distress syndrome, transient tachypnea of the newborn, and meconium aspiration syndrome) in the newborn and their related nursing care.

Concepts for Lecture

1. Respiratory distress syndrome: Lack of sufficient surfactant causes labored respirations and increased work at breathing; seen most frequently in premature newborns; nursing care involves administration of surfactant, close assessment, and supportive care if mechanical ventilation is needed. Refer to "Pathophysiology Illustrated: Respiratory Distress Syndrome (RDS)."
2. Transient tachypnea of the newborn (TTNB): Usually results from excess fluid in the lungs; infant breathes normally at birth but develops symptoms of respiratory distress by 4 to 6 hours of age; nursing care involves initiating oxygen therapy and restricting oral feedings until respiratory status improves.
3. Meconium aspiration syndrome: Signs and symptoms of respiratory distress beginning at birth; may depend upon the amount of meconium that is aspirated; nursing care involves vigorous and deep suctioning prior to infant taking its first breath; after initial suctioning and resuscitation efforts, nursing care involves ongoing assessment for signs and symptoms of respiratory distress and supportive care of the infant requiring mechanical ventilation or ECMO.

POWERPOINT SLIDES 28–42

Figure 29–3. Mechanical ventilatory assistance

Figure 29–6. Premature infant under oxygen hood

Table 29–1. Clinical assessments associated with respiratory distress

SUGGESTION FOR CLASSROOM ACTIVITIES

• Discuss the respiratory assessment of an infant in distress. Include cardiac and neurological implications of respiratory distress syndrome. Show students the various types of oxygen monitors used with newborns. Discuss the nursing interventions done with each type of equipment so as to provide a safe care environment.

SUGGESTION FOR CLINICAL ACTIVITIES

- Ask the students to complete "Thinking Critically: Transient Tachypnea of the Newborn (TTNB)" on page 720 of the textbook. In clinical conference, discuss answers with students.

LEARNING OUTCOME 3

Discuss selected metabolic abnormalities (including cold stress and hypoglycemia), their effects on the newborn, and the nursing implications.

Concepts for Lecture

1. Cold stress sets up the chain of physiologic events of hypoglycemia, pulmonary vasoconstriction, hyperbilirubinemia, respiratory distress, and metabolic acidosis.
2. Nursing interventions include: Keep infant warmed during any transport; observe for any signs of hypoglycemia; have the infant go to breast or feed early in neonatal period; assess blood glucose frequently.

POWERPOINT SLIDES 43–51

Figure 29–7. Cold stress chain of events

Figure 29–8. Potential sites for heel sticks

SUGGESTION FOR CLASSROOM ACTIVITIES

- Discuss how surfactant production is impacted by cold stress. Discuss how heat loss can be blocked in the nursery.

SUGGESTION FOR CLINICAL ACTIVITIES

- Have students review "Skill 10–1: Performing a Capillary Puncture" in the *Clinical Skills Manual*. Allow students to ask questions after reviewing the skill. Ask them to list the nursing considerations when performing a capillary puncture on an infant.

LEARNING OUTCOME 4

Explain the causes, pathophysiology, risks for developing, possible sequelae, clinical therapy, and the difference between physiologic and pathologic jaundice in determining the hospital and community-based nursing care management of the infant with jaundice.

Concepts for Lecture

1. Physiologic jaundice: Occurs in 50% of all newborns; appears after 24 hours of age; not visible after 10 days of age; may require phototherapy.
2. Pathologic jaundice: Usually caused by ABO or Rh incompatibility; jaundice may be present at birth; treatment begins with phototherapy but may progress to exchange transfusions; untreated hyperbilirubinemia (due to either type of jaundice) may result in neurotoxicity.

POWERPOINT SLIDES 52–57

SUGGESTION FOR CLASSROOM ACTIVITIES

- Ask students to research kernicterus on *www.medlineplus.gov*. In small groups, have them discuss warning signs of kernicterus and the nursing role in preventing this health concern.

SUGGESTION FOR CLINICAL ACTIVITIES

- Assign students to research protocol at their clinical site on exchange transfusions and compare the protocol to the clinical position from AWHONN (2005).

LEARNING OUTCOME 5

Explain how Rh incompatibility or ABO incompatibility can lead to the development of hyperbilirubinemia.

Concepts for Lecture

1. Rh incompatibility: Maternal antibodies enter the fetal circulation, then attach to and destroy fetal red blood cells; fetal system produces more RBCs; hyperbilirubinemia, anemia, and jaundice result.
2. ABO incompatibility: Mother is type O and infant is type A or B; less severe than Rh incompatibility.

LEARNING OUTCOME 6

Identify nursing responsibilities and rationale in caring for the newborn receiving phototherapy.

Concepts for Lecture

1. Nursing responsibilities for the newborn receiving phototherapy include: Expose maximum amount of skin surface for optimal therapeutic results; apply eye patches while phototherapy is in progress; assess eyes for signs/symptoms of conjunctivitis every 8 hours; frequently monitor temperature; offer infant water and formula frequently to assist in excretion of bilirubin; keep the parents informed of need for phototherapy and encourage the parents to hold and care for the infant while undergoing phototherapy.

 POWERPOINT SLIDES 58–60

 SUGGESTION FOR CLASSROOM ACTIVITIES

- When discussing hemolytic disease of the newborn, discuss exchange transfusion, erythroblastosis fetalis, and hydrops fetalis.

 SUGGESTION FOR CLINICAL ACTIVITIES

- Ask each student to research hemolytic disease in the newborn and to develop a teaching brochure for expectant parents about its prevention.

 POWERPOINT SLIDES 61–69

Figure 29–11. Infant receiving phototherapy

Figure 29–12. Newborn on fiberoptic "bili" mattress and under phototherapy lights

Teaching Highlights: Instructional checklist for in-room phototherapy

 VIDEO CLIPS

Nursing in Action: Infant Receiving Phototherapy

 SUGGESTIONS FOR CLASSROOM ACTIVITIES

- Ask students to develop a nursing care plan with one physical and one psychosocial nursing diagnoses for a newborn receiving phototherapy.
- Have students watch the video "Nursing in Action: Infant Receiving Phototherapy."

SUGGESTION FOR CLINICAL ACTIVITIES

- Show students equipment needed for phototherapy in the newborn nursery and "bili" mattress. Review a physician's orders for phototherapy.

Learning Outcome 7

Explain the causes and nursing care of infants with anemia or polycythemia.

Concepts for Lecture

1. Anemia in newborns results from prenatal blood loss, birth trauma, infection, or blood group incompatibility. Nursing assessments for signs and symptoms of anemia include recording all amounts of blood taken during laboratory testing.
2. Polycythemia may result from delayed cord clamping, twin-to-twin transfusion, or chronic intrauterine hypoxia: Nursing assessments for signs and symptoms of polycythemia include initial screening of newborn's hematocrit value on admission to nursery.

Learning Outcome 8

Describe the nursing assessments that would lead the nurse to suspect newborn sepsis and the nursing care of the newborn with an infection.

Concepts for Lecture

1. The most common signs of newborn sepsis include: Lethargy or irritability; pallor or duskiness; hypothermia; feeding intolerance; hyperbilirubinemia; tachycardia, bradycardia, or apneic spells.

PowerPoint Slides 70–77

Suggestion for Classroom Activities

- Discuss recombinant human erythropoietin (rEPO) in the newborn and nursing implications. Discuss iron supplementations and nursing implications. Bring examples of iron-fortified formulas to class.

Suggestion for Clinical Activities

- Ask students to research exchange transfusions in newborns on *www.medlineplus.gov*. Have your clinical group develop a nursing problem list in order of priority for a child receiving an exchange transfusion.

PowerPoint Slides 78–82

Table 29–4. Neonatal sepsis antibiotic therapy

Suggestions for Classroom Activities

- Discuss the laboratory tests that are done when sepsis is suspected in a newborn.
- Discuss the laboratory tests that are done when a newborn has an infection.

Suggestion for Clinical Activities

- Have students develop a nursing care plan for the infant experiencing sepsis neonatorum. As a group, discuss nursing interventions for the infant with sepsis and teaching needs of the family.

LEARNING OUTCOME 9

Relate the consequences of maternally transmitted infections, such as maternal syphilis, gonorrhea, herpesviridae family (HSV or CMV), and chlamydia, to the nursing care of infants in the neonatal period.

Concepts for Lecture

1. All infants receive eye prophylaxis with ophthalmic antibiotic. Discuss protocols for neonatal sepsis antibiotic therapy (Table 29–4). Maternal syphilis requires that the infant be isolated from other newborns and receive antibiotics at birth. Maternal herpesvirus infection requires administration of IV antiviral medications in the immediate newborn period as well as multiple cultures (skin, spinal fluid) for presence of herpesvirus.

 POWERPOINT SLIDES 83–95

Table 29–3. Maternally transmitted newborn infections

Table 29–4. Neonatal sepsis antibiotic therapy

 SUGGESTION FOR CLASSROOM ACTIVITIES

- Ask students to research one of the maternally transmitted newborn infections listed in Table 29–3. Have each student give a 5-minute report on the infection that they researched.

 SUGGESTION FOR CLINICAL ACTIVITIES

- Have students develop a nursing care map related to providing supportive care to an infant with sepsis. Have the clinical group discuss how a nurse can create a safe care environment for the infant with sepsis.

LEARNING OUTCOME 10

Describe the interventions to facilitate parental attachment and meet the special initial and long-term needs of parents of at-risk infants.

Concepts for Lecture

1. Assess the parent's level of understanding of the infant's problem. Prepare and facilitate the parents' viewing of the infant. Promote touching and facilitate parental participation in the care of the infant. Facilitate parental adjustment to the infant's special needs. Refer to Figure 29–13.
2. Initially, the parents need to understand the infant's problem, including expected treatments. They need to understand routine well-baby care, how to perform any special procedures needed to care for the infant, referral for normal infant screening procedures, normal growth and development of infants, to have medical follow-up arranged, referral for any special equipment required at home.

 POWERPOINT SLIDES 96–103

Figure 29–13. Parental response patterns during crisis period

Figure 29–15. Beginnings of attachment

Figure 29–16. Facilitating bonding

 SUGGESTIONS FOR CLASSROOM ACTIVITIES

- Discuss factors that may overwhelm parents of an at-risk infant and impact attachment. Discuss therapeutic communication techniques to use with parents. Allow time for students to role-play these techniques.
- Discuss the role of a case manager with parents of at-risk newborns. Discuss the developmental care programs in your community. Discuss the role of the transitional care center with the parents of at-risk newborns.

 SUGGESTIONS FOR CLINICAL ACTIVITIES

- Ask the clinical group to discuss how nurses can improve the self-esteem of parents of at-risk infants. Have the group discuss how culture can impact these parents.
- Ask students to research available community support agencies for families of at-risk newborns in the community. Have them report on these support agencies in a clinical conference.

GENERAL CHAPTER CONSIDERATIONS

1. Have students study and learn key terms listed at beginning of chapter.
2. Have students complete end-of-chapter exercises either in their book or on the MyNursingKit website.
3. Use the Classroom Response Questions provided in PowerPoint to assess students prior to lecture.

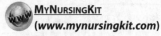

MyNursingKit
(www.mynursingkit.com)

- NCLEX RN® review questions
- Case Studies
- Care Plans
- Critical Concept Review
- Thinking Critically
- Weblinks
- Weblink applications
- Nursing Tools
- Audio Glossary
- Images and Tables Library

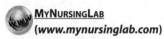

MyNursingLab
(www.mynursinglab.com)

- Knowledge Quick Check
- Pre/Posttests
- Customized study plans
- Images and Tables Library
- *Separate purchase*

CLINICAL SKILLS MANUAL

- *Separate purchase*

PEARSON eTEXT

- Students can search, highlight, take notes, and more all in electronic format
- *Separate purchase*

TESTBANK

CHAPTER 30
POSTPARTAL ADAPTATION AND NURSING ASSESSMENT

LEARNING OUTCOME 1

Describe the basic physiologic changes that occur in the postpartal period as a woman's body returns to its prepregnant state.

Concepts for Lecture

1. The uterus is at the level of the umbilicus within a few hours after childbirth. It decreases by about one finger breadth per day. Placental site heals by a process of exfoliation, so no scar formation occurs. Lochia flow progresses from rubra to serosa to alba.
2. Ovarian function and menstruation return in approximately 6 to 12 weeks in the nonlactating mother. Breasts begin milk production.
3. Intestines are sluggish for a few days—leading to constipation, but return to prepregnant state within a week.
4. Postpartum diuresis occurs—bladder tone is decreased, and takes approximately 6 weeks for the bladder to return to the prepregnant state. A higher than usual boggy uterus deviates to the side, usually indicating a full bladder.
5. Bradycardia is normal for the first 6 to 10 days. Hemostatic system reaches prepregnant state in 3 to 4 weeks. WBC count is often elevated. Activation of clotting factors predisposes to thrombus formation.

 POWERPOINT SLIDES 21–32

Figure 30–1. Involution of the uterus

Figure 30–2. Displacement and deviation of the uterus

 VIDEO CLIPS
Postpartum Assessment

 VIDEO CLIPS
Nursing in Action: Postpartum Assessment

 SUGGESTION FOR CLASSROOM ACTIVITIES

• Incorporate "Skill 4–1: Assessing the Uterine Fundus Following Vaginal Birth" from the *Clinical Skills Manual* into the lecture. Discuss how physiologic adaptation of pregnancy is reversed in the postpartum period.

 SUGGESTIONS FOR CLINICAL ACTIVITIES

• In clinical conference, ask each student the expected height of her/his assigned client's fundus. Assist each student in assessing the uterine fundus on their postpartum clients.
• Have students review the "Postpartum Assessment" videos on *mynursingkit.com*

LEARNING OUTCOME 2

Describe the psychologic adjustments that normally occur during the postpartal period.

Concepts for Lecture

1. Psychologic adjustments include taking in, taking hold, maternal role attainment, and the possibility of postpartum blues.

 POWERPOINT SLIDES 33–37

 SUGGESTION FOR CLASSROOM ACTIVITIES

• Describe the psychologic adjustments of a new mother. Discuss how the nurse can assist the mother in these psychologic adjustments.

 SUGGESTION FOR CLINICAL ACTIVITIES

• Ask students to determine if their assigned clients are in the "taking in" or "taking hold" stage.

LEARNING OUTCOME 3

Explain the components and methods of a systematic postpartal assessment.

Concepts for Lecture

1. Systematic postpartal assessment includes monitoring vital signs; breast examination; assessment of fundus, incision episiotomy, and perineum; assessment of lochia in terms of type, quantity, and characteristics; assessment of bladder and bowels; and assessment of lower extremities. Psychologic assessment components include the expected phase of adjustment to parenthood; the expected level of attachment to the infant; and client education concerning self-care.

LEARNING OUTCOME 4

Describe the normal characteristics and common concerns of the mother considered in a postpartal assessment.

Concepts for Lecture

1. The nurse will often be asked about these common postpartal concerns:
   • A gush of blood that sometimes occurs when the woman first arises
   • Passing clots
   • Night sweats
   • After pains
   • "Large stomach" after birth and failure to lose all the weight gained during pregnancy
2. See Table 30-3 for explanations of these common postpartal concerns.

POWERPOINT SLIDES 38–44

SUGGESTION FOR CLASSROOM ACTIVITIES

• Use the following skills from the *Clinical Skills Manual* in the lecture: "Evaluating Lochia" and "Postpartum Perineal Assessment." Assign "Case Study: Woman Recovering from Cesarean Birth" on *mynursingkit.com* for homework.

SUGGESTION FOR CLINICAL ACTIVITIES

• Assist students in assessing lochia on their assigned clients. Encourage them to distinguish between scant, light, moderate, and heavy. Discuss with students the "Critical Thinking in Action" case study in clinical conference.

POWERPOINT SLIDES 45–47

Figure 30–3. Diastasis recti abdominis

Table 30–3. Common postpartal concerns

SUGGESTION FOR CLASSROOM ACTIVITIES

• Assign students to bring old clothes and a mat to class. Review Figure 30-3. Describe diastasis recti abdominis. Lead class in abdominal strengthening exercises.

SUGGESTIONS FOR CLINICAL ACTIVITIES

• Assign students to review the National Patient Safety Goals.
• In clinical conference, ask students to describe safety concerns with postpartal diaphoresis.

LEARNING OUTCOME 5

Examine the physical and developmental tasks that the mother must accomplish during the postpartal period.

Concepts for Lecture

1. The woman's physical condition returns to a nonpregnant state and she gains competence and confidence in herself as a parent.

POWERPOINT SLIDES 48–49

SUGGESTIONS FOR CLASSROOM ACTIVITIES

- Discuss the developmental tasks of a new mother.
- Have students search the Web to find information concerning the Newborns' and Mothers' Health Protection Act (NMHPA). Allow time in class to discuss the implications of this legislation.

SUGGESTIONS FOR CLINICAL ACTIVITIES

- Have students observe or assist with discharge teaching, including maternal and infant care.
- Arrange for students to attend a meeting of the La Leche League or other postpartum support group. Have students note concerns expressed by the mothers, as well as the purpose and general atmosphere of the meeting. Allow time to share their observations.

LEARNING OUTCOME 6

Explain the factors that influence the development of parent-infant attachment in the nursing assessment of early attachment.

Concepts for Lecture

1. Parent-infant attachment is influenced by the involvement with the woman's own family, stability of relationships and home environment, mother's ability to trust, mother's level of self-esteem, mother's ability to enjoy herself, mother's knowledge of expectations of childbearing and childrearing, and positive reactions to the present pregnancy.

POWERPOINT SLIDES 50–56

Figure 30–5. Engrossment

SUGGESTION FOR CLASSROOM ACTIVITIES

- Discuss the en face position with the students. Describe engrossment in fathers and discuss ways to help them feel more involved with the new baby.

SUGGESTION FOR CLINICAL ACTIVITIES

- Assign students to complete mother-infant bonding activities on *mynursingkit.com*. Ask students to describe the benefits of the en face position with the infant of their assigned mother. Review key elements of reciprocity and ask students if they observed these elements in their assigned mother and infant.

GENERAL CHAPTER CONSIDERATIONS

1. Have students study and learn key terms listed at beginning of chapter.
2. Have students complete end-of-chapter exercises either in their book or on the MyNursingKit website.
3. Use the Classroom Response Questions provided in PowerPoint to assess students prior to lecture.

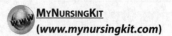

MyNursingKit
(www.mynursingkit.com)

- NCLEX RN® review questions
- Case Studies
- Care Plans
- Critical Concept Review
- Thinking Critically
- Weblinks
- Weblink applications
- Nursing Tools
- Audio Glossary
- Images and Tables Library

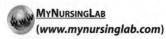

MyNursingLab
(www.mynursinglab.com)

- Knowledge Quick Check
- Pre/Posttests
- Customized study plans
- Images and Tables Library
- *Separate purchase*

CLINICAL SKILLS MANUAL

- *Separate purchase*

PEARSON eTEXT

- Students can search, highlight, take notes, and more all in electronic format
- *Separate purchase*

TESTBANK

CHAPTER 31
THE POSTPARTAL FAMILY: EARLY CARE NEEDS AND HOME CARE

LEARNING OUTCOME 1

Formulate nursing diagnoses and nursing care based on the findings of the "normal" postpartum assessment and teaching needs.

Concepts for Lecture

1. Nursing diagnoses focus on the normal and expected postpartal course.
2. Nursing diagnoses allow the nurse to identify expected outcomes and selected nursing interventions that will help the family meet the expected outcomes and achieve optimal health promotion.
3. The nurse should discuss desired outcomes with the mother and family members.

LEARNING OUTCOME 2

Discuss nursing interventions to promote maternal comfort and well-being.

Concepts for Lecture

1. The nurse can promote and restore maternal physical well-being by monitoring uterine status, vital signs, cardiovascular status, elimination patterns, nutritional needs, sleep and rest, and support and educational needs.
2. In addition, the postpartum woman may need medications to promote comfort, treat anemia, provide immunity to rubella, and prevent development of antigens (in the nonsensitized Rh-negative woman).

LEARNING OUTCOME 3

Explain factors that affect postpartal family wellness in the provision of nursing care and client teaching.

 POWERPOINT SLIDES 20–24

 SUGGESTIONS FOR CLASSROOM ACTIVITIES

- Assign students to complete and submit NCLEX review questions for this chapter on *mynursingkit.com*
- Review the clinical pathway for the postpartal period with the class.

 SUGGESTION FOR CLINICAL ACTIVITIES

- Have students assess a postpartum client and then develop a list of nursing diagnoses in order of priority.

 POWERPOINT SLIDES 25–35

Figure 31–1. Sitz bath

Table 31–2. Essential information for common postpartum drugs

 SUGGESTION FOR CLASSROOM ACTIVITIES

- Identify specific pharmacologic agents used for comfort and sleep (see Table 31–2). Discuss the rationale for RhoGAM and rubella vaccine. Review the nursing implications for the previously mentioned medications. Ask students to list what the clients need to know about their prescribed medications.

 SUGGESTIONS FOR CLINICAL ACTIVITIES

- Provide nursing care for client from delivery, through the recovery period, and into the postpartum period.
- Have students attend a postpartum discharge class. Have them note the questions, behaviors, and responses of the class participants.

 POWERPOINT SLIDES 36–41

Concepts for Lecture

1. The nurse should discuss desired outcomes and goals with the mother and family members.
2. The nurse should design interventions to achieve optimal health promotion.

SUGGESTION FOR CLASSROOM ACTIVITIES

- Have students identify expected outcomes for the physical and psychosocial needs experienced by the mother and her family during the postpartum period.

SUGGESTION FOR CLINICAL ACTIVITIES

- Have students develop a realistic and measurable goal for one physical and one psychosocial goal for their postpartum clients.

LEARNING OUTCOME 4

Compare the postpartal nursing needs of the woman who experienced a cesarean birth with the needs of a woman who gave birth vaginally.

Concepts for Lecture

1. The woman who experiences a cesarean birth has all the needs of the woman who had a vaginal birth: Assessment of the fundus, assessment of the breasts, perineal evaluation (may have varicose veins or hemorrhoids from pregnancy), assessment of lochia flow, and assessment of bowel and bladder.
2. After a cesarean birth, the woman needs assessment of the abdomen, incision, and bowel sounds. She should also turn, cough, and deep breathe.
3. After a cesarean birth, the mother will have a greater need for pain medication. She will also have increased fatigue because of the surgical intervention. The mother may need encouragement to interact with the infant.

POWERPOINT SLIDES 42–49

SUGGESTION FOR CLASSROOM ACTIVITIES

- Outline the assessment protocol for a woman who experiences a cesarean birth. Bring perineal care equipment and supplies to class. Demonstrate care measures used for comfort and healing.

SUGGESTION FOR CLINICAL ACTIVITIES

- Have students develop a priority list of the mother's needs after a cesarean birth. Demonstrate how patient-controlled analgesia equipment is "set up." Discuss what is included in patient-controlled analgesia orders.

LEARNING OUTCOME 5

Examine the nursing needs of the childbearing adolescent during the postpartal period.

Concepts for Lecture

1. The nurse should evaluate the adolescent mother in terms of her level of maturity, available support systems, cultural background, and existing knowledge and then plan care accordingly.

POWERPOINT SLIDES 50–52

SUGGESTIONS FOR CLASSROOM ACTIVITIES

- Include local and state resources for adolescent mothers in the lecture. Describe how these resources can be incorporated in the plan of care for an adolescent mother.
- Discuss how the adolescent mother's educational needs can be met during a pregnancy.

SUGGESTION FOR CLINICAL ACTIVITIES

- Assign students to care for an adolescent mother on the birthing unit or to read a case study on an adolescent mother. Develop a nursing care plan addressing the needs of the adolescent mother.

LEARNING OUTCOME 6

Describe possible approaches to sensitive, holistic nursing care for the woman who relinquishes her newborn.

POWERPOINT SLIDES 53–56

Concepts for Lecture

1. The mother who decides to relinquish her baby needs emotional support. She should be able to decide whether to see and hold her baby, and any special request regarding the birth should be honored.

LEARNING OUTCOME 7

Identify teaching topics related to postpartum discharge.

Concepts for Lecture

1. Prior to discharge, the couple should be given any information necessary for the woman to provide appropriate self-care.
2. Parents should have a beginning skill in caring for their newborn and should be familiar with warning signs of possible complications for mother and baby.
3. Printed information is valuable in helping couples deal with questions that may arise at home.

LEARNING OUTCOME 8

Identify the main purposes and components of home visits during the postpartal period.

Concepts for Lecture

1. The main purposes of the home visit are to:
   - Assess the status of the mother and infant.
   - Assess adaptation and adjustment of the family to the new baby.
   - Determine current informational needs.
   - Provide teaching as needed.
   - Use as an opportunity to answer additional questions related to infant care and feeding, and to provide emotional support to the mother and family.
2. The components of the postpartal home visit include:
   - Establish contact with the mother prior to the visit.
   - Identify the purpose and goals of the visit.
   - Establish rapport with the mother.
   - Maintain safety during the visit.
   - Assess the status of the mother, newborn, and family.
   - Reinforce teaching concerning maternal and newborn care.

 SUGGESTION FOR CLASSROOM ACTIVITIES

- Invite a social worker or lawyer to speak to the class on adoption laws in your state, including the procedures to follow when caring for an infant who is to be, adopted. Be sure to include local and state resources for mothers who relinquish their infants.

 SUGGESTION FOR CLINICAL ACTIVITIES

- Have students develop a nursing care plan with one physical and one psychosocial problem for a mother who relinquishes her infant.

 POWERPOINT SLIDES 57–62

Table 31–4. When to contact the primary care provider

 SUGGESTION FOR CLASSROOM ACTIVITIES

- Outline discharge teaching needs for a new mother. Include information on the family's well-being and care of the infant. Compare and contrast recommendations for postpartum education with the discharge protocols in your community's various agencies.

 SUGGESTION FOR CLINICAL ACTIVITIES

- Have students attend a breastfeeding class or an infant care class in the community. Ask students to determine the teaching styles used in the class attended.

 POWERPOINT SLIDES 63–66

 SUGGESTION FOR CLASSROOM ACTIVITIES

- Assign the Critical Thinking in Action section in Chapter 31. Have students answer the questions. Discuss the answers in class.

 SUGGESTION FOR CLINICAL ACTIVITIES

- Assign clinical students to review the section on Discharge Teaching. Ask them how these guidelines can be used in a postpartal home visit.

LEARNING OUTCOME 9

Summarize actions a nurse should take to ensure personal safety as well as fostering a caring relationship during a home visit.

Concepts for Lecture

1. Nurses need to act proactively to maintain their safety when making home visits by exercising reasonable caution and remaining alert to environmental cues.
2. Fostering a caring relationship in the home involves:
   - Evidence of genuineness and empathy.
   - Establishment of trust and rapport.
   - Positive regard for the mother and family.

LEARNING OUTCOME 10

Discuss maternal and family assessment and anticipated progress after birth.

Concepts for Lecture

1. Assess the infant's weight, length, heart rate, head circumference, and any signs of jaundice.
2. Watch the mother feed the baby and discuss any concerns she has about feeding.
3. Reinforce teaching in the following areas:
   - Position and handling
   - Bathing
   - Dressing
   - Temperature assessment
   - Stool and urine
   - Sleep and activity
   - Crying
   - Safety considerations
   - Newborn screening and necessary immunizations
4. Expected maternal assessments:
   - Vital signs (Should be at prepregnancy level.)
   - Weight (Expect weight to be near prepregnancy level at 6 weeks postpartum.)
   - Condition of the breasts
   - Condition of the abdomen, including a healing cesarean incision, if applicable
   - Elimination pattern (Should return to normal by 4 to 6 weeks postpartum.)
   - Lochia (Should progress from lochia rubra to lochia serosa to lochia alba. If not breastfeeding, menstrual pattern should return at 6 weeks postpartum.)
   - Fundus (Fundus should decrease in size one finger breadth per day after the birth of the baby. Uterus should return to normal size by 6 weeks postpartum.)
   - Perineum (Episiotomy and lacerations should show signs of healing.)
5. Family assessment:
   - Bonding (Appropriate demonstration of bonding should be apparent.)
   - Level of comfort (Parents should display appropriate levels of comfort with the infant.)

POWERPOINT SLIDES 67–69

Table 31–5. Fostering a caring relationship

SUGGESTION FOR CLASSROOM ACTIVITIES

- Assign students to develop a list regarding key safety issues when making a home visit.

SUGGESTION FOR CLINICAL ACTIVITIES

- Review Table 31-5 in clinical conference. Ask students to describe empathetic and genuine behavior that they observed others do while providing nursing care.

POWERPOINT SLIDES 70–72

Evidence-Based Nursing: Postpartum Weight Management

Assessment Guide: Postpartal—First Home Visit and Anticipated Progress at 6 Weeks

SUGGESTION FOR CLASSROOM ACTIVITIES

- Assign students to read "Evidence-Based Nursing: Postpartum Weight Management." Ask students to discuss best practices regarding weight management.

SUGGESTION FOR CLINICAL ACTIVITIES

- Assign clinical students to review the Assessment Guide regarding Postpartal Home Visit. Ask students to discuss how they would assess attachment and adjustment to a parental role.

- Siblings are adjusting to new baby
- Parental role adjustment (Parents should be working on division of labor, changes in financial status, communication changes, readjustment of sexual relations, and adjustment to new daily tasks.)
- Contraception (Parents understand need to choose and use a method of contraception.)

LEARNING OUTCOME 11

Delineate interventions to address the common concerns of breastfeeding mothers following discharge.

Concepts for Lecture

1. Common concerns of the breastfeeding mother include:
   - Nipple soreness
   - Cracked nipples
   - Engorgement
   - Plugged ducts
2. Breastfeeding mothers are encouraged to:
   - Nurse frequently
   - Change the infant's position regularly
   - Allow nipples to air dry after breastfeeding

 POWERPOINT SLIDES 73–75

Table 31–6. Common breastfeeding problems and remedies

 SUGGESTIONS FOR CLASSROOM ACTIVITIES

- Review Table 31-6 regarding self-care measures that a nurse can suggest to a women with a breastfeeding problem.
- Divide the class into three groups. Ask each group to develop three to four questions from Table 31-6. Allow each group to ask their classmates the questions that they develop from Table 31-6.

 SUGGESTION FOR CLINICAL ACTIVITIES

- In clinical conference, ask for two students to role play a nurse making a home visit to a new breastfeeding mother with nipple soreness.

LEARNING OUTCOME 12

Describe the assessment and care of the newborn during postpartal home care.

Concepts for Lecture

1. Assess the infant's weight, length, heart rate, head circumference, and any signs of jaundice.
2. Watch the mother feed the baby and discuss any concerns she has about feeding.
3. Reinforce teaching in the following areas:
   - Position and handling
   - Bathing
   - Dressing
   - Temperature assessment
   - Stool and urine
   - Sleep and activity
   - Crying
   - Safety considerations
   - Newborn screening and necessary immunizations

 POWERPOINT SLIDES 76–78

Evidence in Action: Reducing the Risk of SIDS

 SUGGESTIONS FOR CLASSROOM ACTIVITIES

- Demonstrate various newborn holds using a baby model.
- Discuss the Evidence in Action features box regarding SIDS position.

 SUGGESTION FOR CLINICAL ACTIVITIES

- Discuss the pro and cons of various methods of temperature measurement in a newborn.

GENERAL CHAPTER CONSIDERATIONS

1. Have students study and learn key terms listed at beginning of chapter.
2. Have students complete end-of-chapter exercises either in their book or on the MyNursingKit website.
3. Use the Classroom Response Questions provided in PowerPoint to assess students prior to lecture.

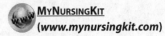

MyNursingKit
(*www.mynursingkit.com*)

- NCLEX RN® review questions
- Case Studies
- Care Plans
- Critical Concept Review
- Thinking Critically
- Weblinks
- Weblink applications
- Nursing Tools
- Audio Glossary
- Images and Tables Library

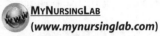

MyNursingLab
(*www.mynursinglab.com*)

- Knowledge Quick Check
- Pre/Posttests
- Customized study plans
- Images and Tables Library
- *Separate purchase*

CLINICAL SKILLS MANUAL

- *Separate purchase*

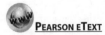

PEARSON eTEXT

- Students can search, highlight, take notes, and more all in electronic format
- *Separate purchase*

TESTBANK

CHAPTER 32
THE POSTPARTAL FAMILY AT RISK

LEARNING OUTCOME 1

Identify the causes of and appropriate nursing interventions for early and late hemorrhage during the postpartal period.

Concepts for Lecture

1. The main causes of postpartum hemorrhage and the appropriate nursing interventions include uterine atony—perform fundal massage and check for clots; laceration of vagina and cervix (suspect if the mother is bleeding heavily in presence of firmly contracted fundus)—contact physician to suture the laceration; retained placental fragments (suspect if the client is bleeding, fundus is firm, and no lacerations are present)—thoroughly inspect placenta; and subinvolution (usually occurs 1 to 2 weeks after birth)—provide mother with discharge instructions, including information about possible complications. Refer to Table 32-1.

POWERPOINT SLIDES 20–25

Table 32–1. Uterine stimulants used to prevent and manage uterine atony

Table 32–2. Signs of postpartal hemorrhage

SUGGESTION FOR CLASSROOM ACTIVITIES

- When discussing uterine atony and fundal massage, ask students to form small groups and ask them to "think ahead" about what nursing assessments need to be made with uterine atony and what equipment may be needed if the woman continues to bleed.

SUGGESTION FOR CLINICAL ACTIVITIES

- In clinical conference, discuss delayed postpartal hemorrhage. Have students "brainstorm" about what clients need to know about this health concern prior to discharge. Review Table 32-1 with clinical students. Question students regarding the nursing implications of uterine stimulants.

LEARNING OUTCOME 2

Develop a nursing care plan that reflects knowledge of etiology, pathophysiology, clinical therapy, nursing and preventive management for the woman experiencing postpartum hemorrhage, reproductive tract infection, urinary tract infection, mastitis, thromboembolic disease, or a postpartal psychiatric disorder.

Concepts for Lecture

1. Nursing care for the postpartal woman experiencing postpartum complications includes obtaining a thorough client prenatal and birth history for any predisposing factors—frequent assessment of all body systems to detect signs and symptoms of complications. These assessments include vital signs, fundal checks, lochial flow, perineum, all incisions, Homan's sign, breast and nipples, and emotional status. Discharge teaching includes ongoing medical management and self-care measures—signs and symptoms of further complications.

POWERPOINT SLIDES 26–34

Table 32–4. Factors associated with development of mastitis

Table 32–6. Measures to decrease risk of thromboembolic disease in childbearing women

SUGGESTIONS FOR CLASSROOM ACTIVITIES

- Ask students to complete the NCLEX-RN® review questions on *mynursingkit.com* for homework and submit them to you.
- Review Tables 32-4 and 32-6. Divide the class into three groups. Assign each group to develop three questions from each table on nursing care and patient teaching.

SUGGESTION FOR CLINICAL ACTIVITIES

- Ask students to discuss risk factors and potential problems of their assigned postpartum clients. Discuss the essential role of the nurse in the prevention of postpartum complications.

LEARNING OUTCOME 3

Evaluate the woman's knowledge of self-care measures, signs of complications to be reported to the primary care provider, and measures to prevent recurrence of complications.

Concepts for Lecture

1. Teaching for self-care includes knowledge of progress of involution; care of the breasts; prevention of infection; expected emotional changes; need for extra rest; nutritional needs; and knowledge of dosage regimens and side effects of prescribed medication. Signs and symptoms of complications include increased vaginal bleeding; fever; foul-smelling vaginal discharge; pain and/or redness in an incision; pain, redness, or swelling in the breasts and/or legs; and overwhelming feelings of sadness or inability to care for the infant.

GENERAL CHAPTER CONSIDERATIONS

1. Have students study and learn key terms listed at beginning of chapter.
2. Have students complete end-of-chapter exercises either in their book or on the MyNursingKit website.
3. Use the Classroom Response Questions provided in PowerPoint to assess students prior to lecture.

 PowerPoint Slides 35–40

Table 32–9. Primary prevention strategies for postpartum depression

 Suggestion for Classroom Activities

- During the lecture, compare local healthcare facilities' postpartum instructions with information from the book. Review Table 32–9. Ask students how they can incorporate postpartum depression primary prevention strategies into discharge instructions.

 Suggestion for Clinical Activities

- Have students develop a teaching-learning handout for a postpartum client on home self-care. Have students discuss these plans in clinical conferences. The following week in client conference, the students should be prepared to present the plan to a client preparing for discharge.

 MyNursingKit
(www.mynursingkit.com)

- NCLEX RN® review questions
- Case Studies
- Care Plans
- Critical Concept Review
- Thinking Critically
- Weblinks
- Weblink applications
- Nursing Tools
- Audio Glossary
- Images and Tables Library

 MyNursingLab
(www.mynursinglab.com)

- Knowledge Quick Check
- Pre/Posttests
- Customized study plans
- Images and Tables Library
- *Separate purchase*

Clinical Skills Manual

- *Separate purchase*

 Pearson eText

- Students can search, highlight, take notes, and more all in electronic format
- *Separate purchase*

 Testbank

CHAPTER 33
GROWTH AND DEVELOPMENT

LEARNING OUTCOME 1

Describe major theories of development as formulated by Freud, Erikson, Piaget, Kohlberg, social learning theorists, and behaviorists.

Concepts for Lecture

1. Freud believed that early childhood experiences form the unconscious motivation for action later in life, and that sexual energy is centered in specific parts of the body at certain ages. Unresolved conflict at a certain stage leads to a fixation of development at that stage.
2. Erikson described eight stages of psychosocial development that occur from birth through old age. When needs are met at each stage, healthy development occurs and the individual moves on to future stages. When needs are not met, an unhealthy outcome occurs that will influence future social relationships.
3. Piaget believed that the child's view of the world is influenced largely by age, experience, and maturational ability. This theory focuses on cognitive (or intellectual) development.
4. Kohlberg developed a framework for understanding moral reasoning. He describes three levels of moral reasoning. Although he also provided age guidelines, many people never reach the highest stage of development.
5. Social learning theorists believe that children learn attitudes, beliefs, and customs through social contact with adults and other children. Children model the behavior they see, and if the behavior is positively reinforced then they tend to repeat it.
6. Behaviorists believe that behaviors can be elicited by positive reinforcement and extinguished by negative reinforcement.

POWERPOINT SLIDES 19–30

Table 33–3. Nursing applications of theories of Freud, Erikson, and Piaget

SUGGESTION FOR CLASSROOM ACTIVITIES

- Divide students into groups and assign each group a developmental theory. Have each group discuss how pediatric nurses can apply that particular theory to nursing practice. Have each group share their findings with the class. (HINT: Nursing applications for each developmental theory are discussed in the text after the theory is described, as well as in Table 33-3.)

SUGGESTION FOR CLINICAL ACTIVITIES

- When caring for children in the clinical setting, have students analyze a child's development using several of the theories discussed in this chapter.

LEARNING OUTCOME 2

Recognize risks developmental progression and factors that protect against those risks.

Concepts for Lecture

1. Based on the concepts of resiliency, families have both protective factors and risk factors. These factors can impact a child's development.

POWERPOINT SLIDES 31–33

Table 33–9. Assessment questions to determine resilience capability

SUGGESTION FOR CLASSROOM ACTIVITIES

- Ask students to list risk factors and protective factors in their own family before discussing this content. Use their answers as a framework for discussion.

SUGGESTION FOR CLINICAL ACTIVITIES

- Have students use Table 33-9, "Assessment Questions to Determine Resilience Capability," to assess a family for protective and risk factors.

Learning Outcome 3

Plan nursing interventions for children that are appropriate for the child's developmental state, based on theoretical frameworks.

Concepts for Lecture

1. Theoretical frameworks of development help pediatric nurses guide their interventions for children based on the child's developmental stage.

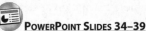
POWERPOINT SLIDES 34–39

SUGGESTION FOR CLASSROOM ACTIVITIES

- Choose a disease that goes across the lifespan (such as pneumonia or fractures) that the students are already familiar with. Use this disease as a basis for class discussion on how nursing interventions would vary based on the child's development (such as giving a nebulizer treatment in an infant versus a toddler versus an adolescent).

SUGGESTION FOR CLINICAL ACTIVITIES

- Invite a child life specialist to speak to the students at a clinical conference about developmentally appropriate activities that pediatric nurses can use while caring for hospitalized children.

Learning Outcome 4

Explain contemporary developmental approaches such as temperament theory, ecologic theory, and the resilience framework.

Concepts for Lecture

1. Ecologic theory emphasizes the presence of mutual interactions between the child (who is unique) and various settings. Neither nature nor nurture is considered of more importance. The levels and systems described in this theory are depicted in Figure 33-3.
2. Temperament theory categorizes children into three patterns of temperament, which can be used to assist in adaptation of the child's environment and for a better understanding of the child. The three patterns include "easy," "difficult," and "slow-to-warm-up."
3. Resilience is the ability to function with healthy responses, even when faced with significant stress and adversity. Resiliency theory states that all individuals experience crises that lead to adaptation and development of inner strengths and the ability to handle future crises.

POWERPOINT SLIDES 40–47

Figure 33–3. Ecologic theory

Table 33–5. Nine parameters of personality

Table 33–6. Patterns of temperament

Learning Outcome 5

Recognize major developmental milestones for infants, toddlers, preschoolers, school-age children, and adolescents.

Concepts for Lecture

1. Infancy is a time of rapid growth and change. The birth weight usually doubles by about 5 months and triples by a year. *Major developmental milestones are reviewed in Tables 33-11 and 33-12.*
2. Toddlers typically display independence and negativism, and they are proud when accomplishing new things. The rate of growth slows during this time, and toddlers often have decreased food intake. By 2 years, the birth weight has usually quadrupled and the child is about one-half of the adult height. *Major developmental milestones are reviewed in Tables 33-13, 33-14, and 33-15.*

POWERPOINT SLIDES 48–58

Table 33–11. Physical growth and development milestones during infancy

Table 33–12. Psychosocial development during infancy

Table 33–13. Growth and development milestones during toddlerhood

Table 33–14. Psychosocial development during toddlerhood

Table 33–15. Communicating with a toddler

3. Preschoolers learn a great deal from the social contact they receive. They develop good language skills and tend to be very busy with projects and tasks. Physical skills and writing ability also increase. *Major developmental milestones are reviewed in Tables 33-16, 33-17, and 33-18.*

4. School-age children are very industrious and begin to find activities that they enjoy and excel in. Peers are beginning to become important, and children develop a sense of achievement and self-esteem. *Major developmental milestones are reviewed in Tables 33-19 and 33-20.*

5. Adolescence marks a time of passage between childhood and adulthood, and teenagers are in a period of identity formation. Puberty occurs during this stage, as does rapid change in growth. Teenagers become interested in new activities and are less dependent on parents for transportation, and peers are important. *Major developmental milestones are reviewed in Tables 33-21 and 33-22.*

Table 33–16. Physical growth and development milestones during the preschool years

Table 33–17. Characteristics of preoperational thought

Table 33–18. Psychosocial development during the preschool years

Table 33–19. Physical growth and development milestones during the school-age years

Table 33–20. Psychosocial development during the school-age years

Table 33–21. Physical growth and development milestones during adolescence

Table 33–22. Psychosocial development during adolescence

VIDEO CLIPS

Growth and Development

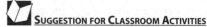

SUGGESTION FOR CLASSROOM ACTIVITIES

- Have students trace their own development from birth through adolescence, identifying as many developmental milestones as possible. For example, students can identify when they said their first words, crawled, walked, and so on. You can ask students to create a timeline or to bring in photographs of the milestones.

SUGGESTION FOR CLINICAL ACTIVITIES

- Require students to complete an assessment of growth and development on each child they care for during their clinical rotation. This assessment can be incorporated into their care plan for that child at *mynursingkit.com*

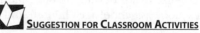

POWERPOINT SLIDES 59–61

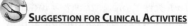

SUGGESTION FOR CLASSROOM ACTIVITIES

- Discuss assessment tools and methods that can be used to gather data from each of the categories of assessment discussed in this objective.

SUGGESTION FOR CLINICAL ACTIVITIES

- Review communication strategies for sharing information and asking questions for each developmental stage. Use a test or procedure, such as drawing blood or starting an IV, as a common framework.

LEARNING OUTCOME 6

Synthesize information from several theoretical approaches to plan assessments of the child's physical growth and developmental milestones.

Concepts for Lecture

1. By using various developmental theories, the nurse can assess the child's growth and development holistically.

Learning Outcome 7

Describe the role of play in the growth and development of children.

Concepts for Lecture

1. Play has often been described as the "work of childhood," and play contributes to the growth and development of children. Play can be described in terms of both social interaction and physical development of gross and fine motor skills.

 POWERPOINT SLIDES 62–68

 SUGGESTION FOR CLASSROOM ACTIVITIES

- Ask students to think about the potential ramifications of children who are not allowed to play (such as children raised in orphanages). How is development affected?

 SUGGESTION FOR CLINICAL ACTIVITIES

- Encourage students to take children they are caring for to the hospital playroom. If the child is in isolation, have the student bring toys to the child's room. By observing children at play, the student will be able to assess many components of growth and development.

Learning Outcome 8

Use data collected during developmental assessments to implement activities that promote development of children and adolescents.

Concepts for Lecture

1. Nursing interventions should be tailored to the child's developmental stage based on data obtained from a holistic assessment.

 POWERPOINT SLIDES 69–72

 SUGGESTION FOR CLASSROOM ACTIVITIES

- Assign students to complete the "NCLEX-RN® Review" questions available on *mynursingkit.com*

 SUGGESTION FOR CLINICAL ACTIVITIES

- During postconference, ask students to think of an example of how they adapted their nursing care based on a child's development level.

GENERAL CHAPTER CONSIDERATIONS

1. Have students study and learn key terms listed at beginning of chapter.
2. Have students complete end-of-chapter exercises either in their book or on the MyNursingKit website.
3. Use the Classroom Response Questions provided in PowerPoint to assess students prior to lecture.

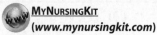

MyNursingKit
(www.mynursingkit.com)

- NCLEX RN® review questions
- Case Studies
- Care Plans
- Critical Concept Review
- Thinking Critically
- Weblinks
- Weblink applications
- Nursing Tools
- Audio Glossary
- Images and Tables Library

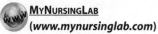

MyNursingLab
(www.mynursinglab.com)

- Knowledge Quick Check
- Pre/Posttests
- Customized study plans
- Images and Tables Library
- *Separate purchase*

CLINICAL SKILLS MANUAL

- *Separate purchase*

PEARSON eTEXT

- Students can search, highlight, take notes, and more all in electronic format
- *Separate purchase*

TESTBANK

Chapter 34
Infant, Child, and Adolescent Nutrition

Learning Outcome 1

Discuss major nutritional concepts pertaining to the growth and development of children.

Concepts for Lecture

1. All children require nutrients in order to grow, but children with conditions such as feeding disorders, food allergies, cystic fibrosis, cerebral palsy, and diabetes have unique nutritional needs.
2. Nutrition monitoring should be provided throughout childhood in order to integrate dietary counseling when needed. Children now live on both ends of the spectrum of nutrition: Those who are hungry and malnourished, and those who are obese.
3. Nutrition and growth require both macronutrients and micronutrients.
4. Dietary Reference Intakes and the Food Guide Pyramid can help families gauge recommended food and caloric intake.

 PowerPoint Slides 22–26

 Video Clips

Nutritional Status

 Suggestion for Classroom Activities

- View "Nutritional Status" video on the *mynursingkit.com* in class. Use this video as a framework for discussing the content in this outcome.

 Suggestion for Clinical Activities

- Have students identify resources in the clinical setting that can be used to help children and families make good dietary choices. These resources may include client education brochures, dietary charts, Web resources, and bulletin boards.

Learning Outcome 2

Describe and plan nursing interventions to meet nutritional needs for all age groups from infancy through adolescence.

Concepts for Lecture

1. During the first year of life, infants progress from taking a few ounces of formula to eating soft table foods. They have extremely high metabolic and growth rates, and triple their birth weight by their first birthday. Breast milk is recommended as the best source of nutrition for infants.
2. Toddlers have much slower metabolic rates than infants, and they often go for long periods of time with little or nothing to eat. This phenomenon is called "physiologic anorexia." Healthy snacks and meals should be provided, and toddlers usually prefer small portions of food. Toddlers should drink milk, but fruit juices should be limited. Toddlers will also begin learning how to eat with others.
3. Preschoolers and toddlers have similar diets, but preschoolers begin to see meals as a social event. They can assist in meal preparation and table setting but need close supervision around sources of heat. Preschoolers may have periods, called *food jags,* where they eat only a few foods for several days or weeks.
4. School-age children grow gradually but eventually have a pre-adolescent growth spurt between 10 and 12 years of age. Children can prepare simple meals and should learn how to choose healthy foods. The loss of deciduous teeth begins at about 6 years of age.

 PowerPoint Slides 27–37

Table 34–2. Introduction of solid foods in infancy

 Video Clips

Breastfeeding and First Foods

 Video Clips

Nursing in Action: Administering a Gavage/Tube Feeding

 Suggestions for Classroom Activities

- Show the video: "Breastfeeding and First Foods" from *mynursingkit.com.* Discuss barriers to breastfeeding that might be encountered by mothers.
- Assign menu planning and nutrition education projects. Have students plan a "Nutrition Teaching Session for Preschoolers" and/or plan a "Two-Day Menu for Vegetarian Teens" for application of the concepts discussed during class. Encourage them to use the Internet for research.

5. Adolescents grow rapidly and require many calories to support growth. Many adolescents prepare much of their own food or eat fast food, and guidance about healthy food choices is important.

LEARNING OUTCOME 3

Integrate methods of nutritional assessment into nursing care of infants, children, and adolescents.

Concepts for Lecture

1. The nutritional status of a child can be assessed by physical measurements (growth) or by dietary intake. Growth can be measured by anthropometric measurements (weight, length, head circumference, etc.) that are then plotted on growth charts.
2. Nutritional status may also be assessed by observing some physical signs and laboratory measurements.
3. Dietary intake can be assessed by 24-hour food recall, food frequency questionnaire, dietary screening history, and food diaries.

LEARNING OUTCOME 4

Discuss common nutritional problems of children growing up in developed countries.

Concepts for Lecture

1. A significant number of children suffer from hunger due to poverty. These children may have *food insecurity,* and often suffer from malnutrition. About 18% of U.S. children live in households that periodically experience food insecurity.
2. Childhood obesity is rapidly escalating due to many factors, including decreased activity, increased television viewing, high levels of dietary fat, snacking, and early menarche. About one-third of American youth are overweight or obese.
3. Children are at risk for foodborne illnesses, and foodborne safety guidelines should be reinforced with families and children.

 SUGGESTION FOR CLINICAL ACTIVITIES

• Have students observe the clinical area and determine how breastfeeding is promoted in the hospital. Are lactation consultants available? Are there posters on the walls from formula companies? Are new mothers given free formula to take home?

 POWERPOINT SLIDES 38–42

Table 34–4 Clinical manifestations of dietary deficiencies/excesses

Table 34–5 Dietary screening history for infants

Table 34–6. Dietary screening history for children

 SUGGESTION FOR CLASSROOM ACTIVITIES

• Make overhead transparencies of growth charts and plot a trend of a child increasing in percentile, decreasing in percentile, and staying the same. Have students discuss possible reasons for these changes in growth over time. Assign "MediaLink Applications: Growth Chart Analysis" activity on *mynursingkit.com* as a method to apply the information discussed during class.

 SUGGESTION FOR CLINICAL ACTIVITIES

• Have students pick one of the four dietary intake tools discussed and administer it to their client. Examples can be found in Tables 34-5 and 34-6. Have students review Skills 9-1 through 9-7 (Growth Measurements) in the *Clinical Skills Manual.*

 POWERPOINT SLIDES 43–51

 VIDEO CLIPS

Children and Overweight

 SUGGESTIONS FOR CLASSROOM ACTIVITIES

• Have students locate and bring to class a recent article in the news or mass media about childhood obesity. Discuss factors relating to the increase in childhood obesity and what nurses can do to influence the problem.
• Show the video "Children and Overweight." Use this video as a way to discuss the differences between being overweight and being obese.

4. Children may have dietary deficiencies of iron, calcium, vitamin D, and folic acid. New recommendations for vitamin D intake and supplementation state that infants and children should receive at least 400 IU of vitamin D daily.

LEARNING OUTCOME 5

Apply the nursing process to care for children with eating disorders.

Concepts for Lecture

1. Children may have numerous eating disorders, including pica, failure to thrive, anorexia nervosa, bulimia, and food allergies.
2. The nursing process will be applied to discuss anorexia nervosa as a model case for children with eating disorders.

 SUGGESTIONS FOR CLINICAL ACTIVITIES

- Students will often encounter obese children who have been admitted to the hospital for an unrelated disorder. Ask students what interventions for obesity can be accomplished during the child's admission.
- How can students teach children about preventing foodborne illnesses? Challenge students to think creatively about how to teach the four components of foodborne safety to children.

 POWERPOINT SLIDES 52–59

 VIDEO CLIPS

Anorexia Nervosa

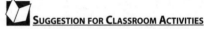 **SUGGESTION FOR CLASSROOM ACTIVITIES**

- Show the video, "Anorexia Nervosa," from *mynursingkit.com*, before discussing the nursing plan for anorexia described above.

SUGGESTION FOR CLINICAL ACTIVITIES

- During clinical conference, ask students to suppose they were caring for a teenager with anorexia. What are some of the challenges they might face? What would they do if a physician ordered treatments (such as nutrition through an NG tube) that the teenager refused? How can the psychiatric components of the disease be addressed in the hospital?

GENERAL CHAPTER CONSIDERATIONS

1. Have students study and learn key terms listed at beginning of chapter.
2. Have students complete end-of-chapter exercises either in their book or on the MyNursingKit website.
3. Use the Classroom Response Questions provided in PowerPoint to assess students prior to lecture.

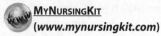

MyNursingKit
(www.mynursingkit.com)

- NCLEX RN® review questions
- Case Studies
- Care Plans
- Critical Concept Review
- Thinking Critically
- Weblinks
- Weblink applications
- Nursing Tools
- Audio Glossary
- Images and Tables Library

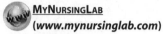

MyNursingLab
(www.mynursinglab.com)

- Knowledge Quick Check
- Pre/Posttests
- Customized study plans
- Images and Tables Library
- *Separate purchase*

CLINICAL SKILLS MANUAL

- *Separate purchase*

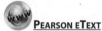

PEARSON eTEXT

- Students can search, highlight, take notes, and more all in electronic format
- *Separate purchase*

TESTBANK

CHAPTER 35
PEDIATRIC ASSESSMENT

LEARNING OUTCOME 1

Describe the elements of a health history for infants and children of different ages.

Concepts for Lecture

1. Client information includes the child's name, nickname, age, gender, and ethnicity. Birth date, address, phone number, and emergency contact information should be obtained as well.
2. Physiologic data includes the chief complaint, history of present illness, past medical and family history, current health status, and review of systems. *Tables 35-1 through 35-3 in the text are excellent references.*
3. Psychosocial data includes the family composition, socioeconomic factors, housing, school, and childcare routines. *Table 35-5 is a good reference.*
4. Developmental data includes information about the child's motor, cognitive, language, and social development.

POWERPOINT SLIDES 26–30

Table 35–1. History of present illness or injury

Table 35–2. Birth history

Table 35–3. Familial or hereditary diseases

Table 35–5. Daily living patterns

SUGGESTION FOR CLASSROOM ACTIVITIES

- Use a case study format to teach this outcome, using a hypothetical child and family to model a thorough history.

SUGGESTION FOR CLINICAL ACTIVITIES

- Early in the clinical rotation, assign students to take health histories for newly admitted clients. This works well on units that receive a lot of admissions while students are present.

LEARNING OUTCOME 2

Identify communication strategies to improve the quality of historical data collected.

Concepts for Lecture

1. Clear communication is very important, as the information collected forms the basis of many decisions. An interpreter should be used if a language barrier exists. Always be honest when answering parents' questions.
2. Techniques that help the nurse to build rapport with a family include introductions, purpose of the interview, privacy, asking open-ended questions, and asking only one question at a time. In addition, the child should be involved in the interview if his or her age is appropriate.
3. Active listening is important in order to accurately interpret the information shared during the interview.
4. Some cultures have different views about eye contact, interaction with healthcare providers, and physical touch.

POWERPOINT SLIDES 31–35

SUGGESTION FOR CLASSROOM ACTIVITIES

- Demonstrate the preceding communication methods to the class by role modeling the techniques with a student volunteer. It may be helpful to perform the demonstrations twice: First using closed communication techniques, then again using the open communication techniques described previously.

SUGGESTION FOR CLINICAL ACTIVITIES

- Identify resources available in the local clinical setting for families from various cultures. What interpreting resources are available and during what hours? What accommodations for cultural food preferences and visitation patterns are allowed?

LEARNING OUTCOME 3

Describe the strategies to gain cooperation of a young child for assessment.

Concepts for Lecture

1. There are several strategies that nurses can use to gain the child's co-operation during the physical examination.

LEARNING OUTCOME 4

Describe the differences in sequence of the physical assessment for infants, children, and adolescents.

Concepts for Lecture

1. The approach and the sequence of the physical examination vary by age. Different strategies can be applied across the lifespan in order to facilitate a stress-free physical exam.

POWERPOINT SLIDES 36–37

SUGGESTION FOR CLASSROOM ACTIVITIES

- Bring a stuffed animal and various assessment tools (e.g., stethoscope, penlight, reflex hammer, etc.) to class so you can demonstrate these strategies during class.

SUGGESTION FOR CLINICAL ACTIVITIES

- Demonstrate the above strategies as you role model performing an assessment on a young child during the first day of clinical.

POWERPOINT SLIDES 38–45

ANIMATION

3D Eye

ANIMATION

Otoscope Examination

ANIMATION

Mouth and Throat Examination

ANIMATION

Movement of Joints

SUGGESTION FOR CLASSROOM ACTIVITIES

- How does the developmental approach to the exam relate to the child's developmental age? For example, why does examining a stuffed animal work well with a preschool child but not well with an adolescent? Encourage students to think about the developmental tasks that children progress through.

SUGGESTION FOR CLINICAL ACTIVITIES

- Encourage students to create a chart that highlights the differences in the sequence and approach to the physical exam as it varies by age. They can use this as a reminder when they assess children of different ages.

LEARNING OUTCOME 5

Modify physical assessment techniques according to the age and developmental stage of the child.

Concepts for Lecture

1. Health assessment begins with first meeting the child, and includes an overview of the child's appearance and behavior. Growth measurements and vital signs are taken at this point.
2. Assessment techniques include inspection, palpation, auscultation, and percussion.
3. Although the physical assessment may have to be adapted based on the developmental level of the child, assessment generally proceeds from head to toe. A systematic approach prevents components of the assessment from being omitted.

 POWERPOINT SLIDES 45–94

Figure 35–3. Tenting of the skin associated with poor skin turgor

Figure 35–5. Inspecting for facial symmetry

Figure 35–6. External structures of the eye

Figure 35–7. Inspecting for palpebral slant

Figure 35–8. Upward palpebral slant

Figure 35–12. Ear placement

Figure 35–20. Palpating the lymph nodes

Figure 35–21. Landmarks of the chest

Figure 35–22. Vertical landmarks of the chest

Figure 35–23. Two types of abnormal chest shape

Figure 35–25. Auscultating heart sounds

Figure 35–26. Topographic landmarks of the abdomen

Figure 35–27. Anatomic structures of the female genital and perineal area

Figure 35–29. Normal stages of breast development

Figure 35–33. Evaluating spinal alignment

Figure 35–34. Inspection of the spine for scoliosis

As Children Grow: Sutures

As Children Grow: Growth and Development of Sinuses

Pathophysiology Illustrated: Tonsil Size with Infection

 SUGGESTIONS FOR CLASSROOM ACTIVITIES

- Make in-class use of the following animations on *mynursingkit.com:* Otoscope Examination Animation, Mouth and Throat Examination Animation, 3D Eye Animation, and Movement of Joints Animation.
- Demonstrate a complete health assessment on an actual child for the class. This usually works well with a school-age child as the model, as long as privacy is respected. Children of faculty members and/or students are often willing to participate.

SUGGESTION FOR CLINICAL ACTIVITIES

- On the first day of the clinical rotation, have students pair up and perform physical assessments on multiple children, including an infant, toddler, preschool or school-age child, and adolescent. This exposes the students to the differences across the pediatric age range. Support and role modeling from the instructor are important for this activity to be successful.

POWERPOINT SLIDES 95–96

LEARNING OUTCOME 6

List five normal variations in pediatric physical findings (such as a Mongolian spot in an infant) found during a physical assessment.

Concepts for Lecture

1. This outcome points out common differences in pediatric assessment findings versus adult assessment findings.

SUGGESTION FOR CLASSROOM ACTIVITIES

- List normal assessment findings across the lifespan on the board, including those discussed in this outcome. Include normal findings not commonly seen in children (e.g., loss of hair) and have students identify which of the normal findings are commonly seen in children.

SUGGESTION FOR CLINICAL ACTIVITIES

- Remind students that the most important assessment skill is to be able to recognize what is normal. If assessment findings are abnormal, emphasize that they should focus on describing their findings rather than putting a name to it.

LEARNING OUTCOME 7

Determine the sexual maturity rating of males and females based upon physical signs of secondary sexual characteristics present.

Concepts for Lecture

1. The age of onset of secondary sexual characteristics varies widely, but does follow a predictable pattern.
2. Females usually begin breast development between 9 and 14 years. Breast development may be asymmetric.
3. The presence, amount, and distribution of pubic hair indicates sexual development in girls. Breast development usually precedes pubic hair development, and the presence of pubic hair before age 8 is unusual.
4. Genital development and the development of pubic hair indicates sexual development in boys. Pubic hair is uncommon before age 9. Boys who have not begun showing development by age 14 should be referred for further evaluation.
5. The sexual maturity rating (SMR) is an average of the breast and pubic hair Tanner stages in females and of the genital and pubic hair stages in males.

POWERPOINT SLIDES 95–105

Figure 35–30. The stages of female pubic hair development with sexual maturation

Figure 35–31. The stages of male pubic hair and external genital development with sexual maturation

SUGGESTION FOR CLASSROOM ACTIVITIES

- Ask students what they would say to a school-age child or adolescent who was concerned about his or her sexual development.

SUGGESTION FOR CLINICAL ACTIVITIES

- Discuss methods the nurse can employ to make genital examination less anxious for children of various ages. How does the approach for a preschooler differ from that of an adolescent?

Learning Outcome 8

Recognize at least five important signs of a serious alteration in health condition that require urgent nursing intervention.

Concepts for Lecture

1. The physical assessment usually offers important findings about a child's health condition. Assessment findings may be subtle or obvious. Continuous monitoring and reassessment to identify trends are critical in identifying serious changes in the child's status.

General Chapter Considerations

1. Have students study and learn key terms listed at beginning of chapter.
2. Have students complete end-of-chapter exercises either in their book or on the MyNursingKit website.
3. Use the Classroom Response Questions provided in PowerPoint to assess students prior to lecture.

  PowerPoint Slides 106–112

 Suggestion for Classroom Activities

- Discuss as a class the general principles that nurses should follow when working with a child who has a sudden change in his or her health status.

 Suggestion for Clinical Activities

- Locate emergency equipment in the clinical setting. If possible, have students practice handling the equipment (examples: connecting an Ambu-bag to oxygen supply, bagging a child, etc.).

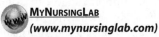 **MyNursingKit**
(www.mynursingkit.com)

- NCLEX RN® review questions
- Case Studies
- Care Plans
- Critical Concept Review
- Thinking Critically
- Weblinks
- Weblink applications
- Nursing Tools
- Audio Glossary
- Images and Tables Library

 MyNursingLab
(www.mynursinglab.com)

- Knowledge Quick Check
- Pre/Posttests
- Customized study plans
- Images and Tables Library
- *Separate purchase*

Clinical Skills Manual

- *Separate purchase*

 Pearson eText

- Students can search, highlight, take notes, and more all in electronic format
- *Separate purchase*

Testbank

CHAPTER 36
HEALTH PROMOTION AND MAINTENANCE: GENERAL CONCEPTS, THE NEWBORN, AND THE INFANT

LEARNING OUTCOME 1

Define health promotion and health maintenance.

Concepts for Lecture

1. *Health promotion* refers to activities that increase well-being or enhance wellness or health. *Health maintenance* refers to activities that preserve a person's present state of health and that prevent disease or injury occurrence.

 POWERPOINT SLIDES 26–29

 SUGGESTION FOR CLASSROOM ACTIVITIES

- To help students understand the difference between health promotion and health maintenance, list several examples of each concept on the chalkboard. Have students identify which examples fit with each concept.

LEARNING OUTCOME 2

Describe how health promotion and health maintenance are addressed by partnering with families during health supervision visits.

Concepts for Lecture

1. Health promotion and health maintenance are integrated into healthcare visits. Nurses partner with families during these visits by involving the family during the information-gathering part of the visit.

 POWERPOINT SLIDES 30–31

 SUGGESTION FOR CLASSROOM ACTIVITIES

- Ask the class how they might collect an accurate health history during a health supervision visit if a relative who did not know the infant well brought the infant to the visit.

LEARNING OUTCOME 3

Describe the components of a health supervision visit.

Concepts for Lecture

1. Key assessments that are completed during health supervision visits include growth and development, physical activity, oral health, mental and spiritual health, and relationships.
2. Disease screening and injury prevention strategies are important components of health supervision visits.

 POWERPOINT SLIDES 32–41

 SUGGESTION FOR CLINICAL ACTIVITIES

- To help students become proficient at using growth charts, require them to plot the height, weight, and body mass index of each infant they care for during their clinical rotation.

LEARNING OUTCOME 4

Explore the nurse's role in providing health promotion and health maintenance for the newborn and infant.

Concepts for Lecture

1. The nurse can integrate six concepts into the care of infants during health maintenance visits.

 POWERPOINT SLIDES 42–43

 SUGGESTION FOR CLASSROOM ACTIVITIES

- Lead students in a discussion of how the six concepts described in this outcome can be applied to actual practice.

LEARNING OUTCOME 5

Describe the general observations made of infants and their families as they come to the pediatric healthcare home for health supervision visits.

Concepts for Lecture

1. The nurse can gather much information by observing the infant and family interact in the waiting room and examination room.

 PowerPoint Slides 44–48

Figure 36–6. General observations

 Suggestion for Classroom Activities

- When showing Figure 36-6, ask the students what observations the nurse could make if he or she saw this family in the waiting room. What further questions would they want to follow up on?

 Suggestion for Clinical Activities

- Arrange for students to work with a pediatric nurse practitioner who cares for infants and their parents in the office setting. Have the student call the infant and parents into the exam room. In postconference, have students discuss findings regarding their observations.

LEARNING OUTCOME 6

Describe the areas of assessment and intervention for health supervision visits of newborns and infants—growth and developmental surveillance, nutrition, physical activity, oral health, mental and spiritual health, family and social relations, disease prevention strategies, and injury prevention strategies.

Concepts for Lecture

1. Because infants grow and change rapidly, health supervision visits occur frequently during this developmental stage.

 PowerPoint Slides 49–59

Table 36–2. Nutrition teaching for health promotion and health maintenance visits

 Suggestion for Classroom Activities

- Many students do not realize how difficult it is to install car seats correctly. Before class, assign students to research how to properly install car seats in order to provide adequate protection during a collision.

 Suggestion for Clinical Activities

- Arrange for students to rotate through a pediatric clinic that performs health supervision visits for infants and toddlers.

LEARNING OUTCOME 7

Plan health promotion and health maintenance strategies employed during health supervision visits of newborns and infants.

Concepts for Lecture

1. Health promotion and health maintenance strategies are routinely employed during health supervision visits.

 PowerPoint Slides 60–61

 Suggestion for Classroom Activities

- Lead students in a discussion about how the strategies discussed in this outcome can help to promote health.

LEARNING OUTCOME 8

Recognize the importance of family in newborn and infant health care, and include family assessment in each health supervision visit.

Concepts for Lecture

1. Because the family is viewed as the expert about the infant, it is critical to involve the family in each health supervision visit.

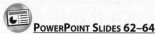
POWERPOINT SLIDES 62–64

SUGGESTION FOR CLASSROOM ACTIVITIES

- Invite parents to speak to the class about their experiences with health supervision visits.

SUGGESTION FOR CLINICAL ACTIVITIES

- Many families do not participate in health supervision visits, and their only opportunity to receive health promotion is when the infant is hospitalized. Identify local resources that the nurse could refer families to in order to receive free or low-cost health supervision visits.

LEARNING OUTCOME 9

Integrate pertinent mental healthcare into health supervision visits for newborns and infants.

Concepts for Lecture

1. An infant's mental health is related to early experiences, inborn characteristics such as temperament and resilience, and relationships with caregivers. Assessment of parent-infant bonding, discussion of separation anxiety, and discussion of self-regulation should be part of the health promotion visit.

POWERPOINT SLIDES 65–70

Figure 36–8. Assessing mental health

SUGGESTION FOR CLASSROOM ACTIVITIES

- Parents often have questions about how to encourage infants to sleep longer at night, so an understanding of infant sleep patterns is important. Have students review "Evidence-Based Nursing: Infant Sleep." Use the Critical Thinking questions as a basis for discussion in class.

LEARNING OUTCOME 10

Synthesize data about the family and other social relationships to promote and maintain health of newborns and infants.

Concepts for Lecture

1. Families are the primary site where the infant learns about socialization and relationships. Therefore, it is important to identify families that have depression, violence, or abuse in order to promote positive socialization in those infants.
2. The infant undergoes significant development during the first year of life that enhances socialization and human relationships.

POWERPOINT SLIDES 71–74

SUGGESTION FOR CLASSROOM ACTIVITIES

- Ask students to think of other issues that may affect the relationships of infants with other people in the baby's life (examples: financial considerations, attending daycare, presence of relatives, etc.).

SUGGESTION FOR CLINICAL ACTIVITIES

- Have students visit the playroom at the hospital to observe infants socializing with other children and adults.

GENERAL CHAPTER CONSIDERATIONS

1. Have students study and learn key terms listed at beginning of chapter.
2. Have students complete end-of-chapter exercises either in their book or on the MyNursingKit website.
3. Use the Classroom Response Questions provided in PowerPoint to assess students prior to lecture.

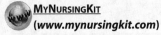

MyNursingKit
(www.mynursingkit.com)

- NCLEX RN® review questions
- Case Studies
- Care Plans
- Critical Concept Review
- Thinking Critically
- Weblinks
- Weblink applications
- Nursing Tools
- Audio Glossary
- Images and Tables Library

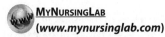

MyNursingLab
(www.mynursinglab.com)

- Knowledge Quick Check
- Pre/Posttests
- Customized study plans
- Images and Tables Library
- *Separate purchase*

CLINICAL SKILLS MANUAL

- *Separate purchase*

PEARSON eTEXT

- Students can search, highlight, take notes, and more all in electronic format
- *Separate purchase*

TESTBANK

CHAPTER 37
HEALTH PROMOTION AND MAINTENANCE: THE TODDLER, THE PRESCHOOLER, AND THE SCHOOL-AGE CHILD

LEARNING OUTCOME 1

Describe the areas of assessment and intervention for health supervision visits for children—growth and developmental surveillance, nutrition, physical activity, oral health, mental and spiritual health, family and social relations, disease prevention strategies, and injury prevention strategies.

Concepts for Lecture

1. Because toddlers and preschoolers grow and change rapidly, health supervision visits occur frequently during this developmental stage. Most providers see children at 12, 15, and 18 months, and at 2, 3, and 4 years of age.
2. School-age children are relatively healthy and require few immunizations, so health supervision visits are typically done at 5, 6, 8, 10, 11, and 12 years of age.

 POWERPOINT SLIDES 26–45

Table 37–1. Nutrition teaching for health promotion and health maintenance visits

 VIDEO CLIPS

Making the Pacifier Decision

 SUGGESTION FOR CLASSROOM ACTIVITIES

- Before class, assign students to research local cases of children who were injured (such as drownings, falls, burns, motor vehicle collisions, etc.). During class, use these cases as a framework to discuss the importance of injury prevention.

 SUGGESTION FOR CLINICAL ACTIVITIES

- Arrange for students to rotate through a pediatric clinic that performs health supervision visits for toddlers and young children. Have students describe activities they observed that relate to health promotion.

LEARNING OUTCOME 2

State components of self-concept for preschool and school-age children.

Concepts for Lecture

1. The major components of self-concept include a sense of accomplishment, positive self-esteem, body image, and sexuality. The school-age years are an important time for the development of a child's self-concept.

 POWERPOINT SLIDES 46–53

 SUGGESTION FOR CLASSROOM ACTIVITIES

- Children often get information about sexuality through the media. Show clips of TV shows, movies, or advertisements that children may see on TV and discuss the information that children may receive from these programs. Prime-time TV and day-time talk shows are a good source of media for this activity.

 SUGGESTION FOR CLINICAL ACTIVITIES

- Assessing a child's self-esteem is an important component of the holistic assessment. Encourage students to use the questions discussed in "Teaching Highlights: Evaluating and Fostering Self-Esteem," during their care of hospitalized children.

LEARNING OUTCOME 3

Plan health promotion and health maintenance strategies employed during health supervision visits of children.

Concepts for Lecture

1. Health promotion and health maintenance strategies are routinely employed during health supervision visits.

LEARNING OUTCOME 4

Discuss the importance of family in child health care, and include family assessment in each health supervision visit.

Concepts for Lecture

- Because the family is viewed as the expert about the child, it is critical to involve the family in each health supervision visit.

LEARNING OUTCOME 5

Integrate pertinent mental healthcare into health supervision visits for children.

Concepts for Lecture

1. Fostering a positive self-image is important to the toddler's and preschooler's mental health. Common mental health concerns in this age group include nightmares, temper tantrums, and daily stressors.
2. School-age children are developing new cognitive skills, and the development of a positive self-concept contributes to mental health in this age group.

 POWERPOINT SLIDES 54–58

 SUGGESTION FOR CLASSROOM ACTIVITIES

- Lead students in a discussion about how the strategies discussed in this outcome can help to promote health.

 SUGGESTION FOR CLINICAL ACTIVITIES

- Encourage students to think about how health promotion topics can be transferred to the care of the hospitalized child. For example, a school-age child who is hospitalized with appendicitis probably rides his bicycle, so it is appropriate for the nurse to take the opportunity to teach about proper use of helmets. This approach helps students think beyond the admitting diagnosis.

 POWERPOINT SLIDES 59–61

 SUGGESTION FOR CLASSROOM ACTIVITIES

- Invite parents to speak to the class about their experiences with health supervision visits.

 SUGGESTION FOR CLINICAL ACTIVITIES

- As students observe health promotion visits, have them compare and contrast different families using a family assessment tool.

 POWERPOINT SLIDES 62–67

 VIDEO CLIPS

Temper Tantrums

 SUGGESTION FOR CLASSROOM ACTIVITIES

- While discussing self-regulation, show the video "Temper Tantrums," available on *mynursingkit.com*

 SUGGESTION FOR CLINICAL ACTIVITIES

- Have students use "Teaching Highlights: Evaluating and Fostering Self-Esteem" to assess a child's self-esteem. This child could be a hospitalized child or a child in the family or community.

Learning Outcome 6

Synthesize data about the family and other social relationships to promote and maintain the health of children.

Concepts for Lecture

1. Toddlers and preschoolers make great strides in relationships and socialization, which are often expressed through play. One of the major goals during this age is to learn to be separate from parents.
2. School-age children are gradually moving away from family as the center of life, and peer groups become more important. Peer pressure can cause children to engage in risky behaviors.

General Chapter Considerations

1. Have students study and learn key terms listed at beginning of chapter.
2. Have students complete end-of-chapter exercises either in their book or on the MyNursingKit website.
3. Use the Classroom Response Questions provided in PowerPoint to assess students prior to lecture.

PowerPoint Slides 68–74

Suggestion for Classroom Activities

- Before class, assign students to research programs in schools that address bullying. Use this information to further discuss the problem of bullying in schools.

Suggestion for Clinical Activities

- Have students visit the playroom at the hospital to observe children playing "side by side" and cooperatively.

MyNursingKit
(www.mynursingkit.com)

- NCLEX RN® review questions
- Case Studies
- Care Plans
- Critical Concept Review
- Thinking Critically
- Weblinks
- Weblink applications
- Nursing Tools
- Audio Glossary
- Images and Tables Library

MyNursingLab
(www.mynursinglab.com)

- Knowledge Quick Check
- Pre/Posttests
- Customized study plans
- Images and Tables Library
- *Separate purchase*

Clinical Skills Manual

- *Separate purchase*

Pearson eText

- Students can search, highlight, take notes, and more all in electronic format
- *Separate purchase*

Testbank

CHAPTER 38
HEALTH PROMOTION AND MAINTENANCE: THE ADOLESCENT

LEARNING OUTCOME 1

Identify the major health concerns of the adolescent years.

Concepts for Lecture

1. The major health concerns of adolescents include school performance, sexual issues, body image issues, and the need for independence.

 POWERPOINT SLIDES 15–18

 SUGGESTION FOR CLASSROOM ACTIVITIES

- Before class, assign students to complete "Case Study: Immunization Update," available on *mynursingkit.com*. Use this activity as a basis for discussing typical reasons that adolescents visit a healthcare provider.

 SUGGESTION FOR CLINICAL ACTIVITIES

- Have students assist with sports examinations for adolescents. This activity works best for summer classes since the majority of sports examinations are done in the late summer before classes begin.

LEARNING OUTCOME 2

Describe the general observations made of adolescents and their families as they come to the pediatric healthcare home for health supervision visits.

Concepts for Lecture

1. Assessment of the adolescent and family begins when the nurse first meets the family in the waiting room, where several important observations are made.

 POWERPOINT SLIDES 19–20

 SUGGESTION FOR CLASSROOM ACTIVITIES

- List several conditions that adolescents may have on the chalkboard (such as skin infections, cough, limp, abdominal pain, etc.) and have students discuss whether parents should come into the examination room with the adolescent. Relate this concept back to the issues of privacy and adolescent development.

 SUGGESTION FOR CLINICAL ACTIVITIES

- Have students suggest elements of waiting rooms that would promote adolescents feeling welcome and comfortable (examples include design elements, activities for teens, and age-appropriate magazines).

LEARNING OUTCOME 3

Apply communication skills to interactions with adolescents and their families.

 POWERPOINT SLIDES 21–24

Concepts for Lecture

1. Adolescents need their parents for guidance and reassurance as the teenager strives to gain independence. Adolescents commonly strike out at parents, test limits, and have conflicts with their parents. There are several communication skills that can be used to promote positive interactions between adolescents and their families.

SUGGESTIONS FOR CLASSROOM ACTIVITIES

- Have students provide examples of the communication strategies discussed in this outcome.
- Have students role play how the communication strategies described can be applied. Have one or two students play the role of the parents and another student play the role of the adolescent. This activity works better if you provide the students with cue cards about what the situation is and what you would like their responses to be.

SUGGESTION FOR CLINICAL ACTIVITIES

- Invite a social worker or child-life specialist from the hospital to speak with students during clinical conference about communication strategies for adolescents and parents.

LEARNING OUTCOME 4

Apply assessment skills to plan data-gathering methods for nutrition, physical activity, and mental health status of youth.

Concepts for Lecture

1. Nutrition can be a challenge for many adolescents, as they often have poor diets. Weight changes may also be a concern. After assessing nutritional status, the nurse can suggest several ways to promote a healthy diet.
2. Physical activity tends to decrease during adolescence, especially among girls. Promoting physical activity is important, as it sets up habits for lifelong exercise and activity.
3. Adolescents often have challenges with mental health issues, which are closely linked to developmental tasks such as independence, forming close relationships, gaining confidence, and setting goals for the future.

POWERPOINT SLIDES 25–33

VIDEO CLIPS

Teen Mental and Spiritual Health

SUGGESTION FOR CLASSROOM ACTIVITIES

- Before discussing mental health during adolescence, show the video "Teen Mental and Spiritual Health," available on *mynursingkit.com*. Use this video as a basis for the discussion.

SUGGESTION FOR CLINICAL ACTIVITIES

- When caring for a hospitalized adolescent, have students note what the adolescent is eating on his or her meal tray. This can often open the door for a discussion about health nutrition during adolescence.

LEARNING OUTCOME 5

Synthesize data from history and examination of adolescent and family with knowledge of adolescent development to plan approaches useful with the family during health supervision visits.

Concepts for Lecture

1. The adolescent is still growing and developing, so it is important to monitor and plot growth. Major developmental tasks during adolescence involve the adolescent separating from family and establishing positive peer relationships.

POWERPOINT SLIDES 34–37

SUGGESTION FOR CLASSROOM ACTIVITIES

- Create several data sets of height and weight for various ages of adolescents. During class, have students plot height, weight, and BMI on growth charts using the data you supply.

SUGGESTION FOR CLINICAL ACTIVITIES

- Ask students to practice plotting height, weight, and BMI on adolescents they care for during clinical.

LEARNING OUTCOME 6

Intervene with adolescents by integrating activities to promote health and to prevent disease and injury.

Concepts for Lecture

1. Although most adolescents are generally healthy, there are several screening tests that should be performed during adolescence.
2. Injury is the greatest health hazard for adolescents, so injury prevention is a critical topic to discuss during health visits with adolescents. *Tables 38-3 and 38-4 are good references for this content.*

GENERAL CHAPTER CONSIDERATIONS

1. Have students study and learn key terms listed at beginning of chapter.
2. Have students complete end-of-chapter exercises either in their book or on the MyNursingKit website.
3. Use the Classroom Response Questions provided in PowerPoint to assess students prior to lecture.

 POWERPOINT SLIDES 38–44

Table 38–3. Injury prevention in adolescence

Table 38–4. Injury prevention topics for adolescents

 SUGGESTION FOR CLASSROOM ACTIVITIES

- Before class, assign students to complete the activity, "Weblink Applications: Develop a Teaching Plan: Smoking Education," available on *mynursingkit.com*. Use this activity as a framework for discussing disease prevention among adolescents.

 SUGGESTION FOR CLINICAL ACTIVITIES

- Have students identify resources available in the local clinical setting that can be used to teach adolescents about disease and injury prevention strategies.

 MYNURSINGKIT (*www.mynursingkit.com*)

- NCLEX RN® review questions
- Case Studies
- Care Plans
- Critical Concept Review
- Thinking Critically
- Weblinks
- Weblink applications
- Nursing Tools
- Audio Glossary
- Images and Tables Library

 MYNURSINGLAB (*www.mynursinglab.com*)

- Knowledge Quick Check
- Pre/Posttests
- Customized study plans
- Images and Tables Library
- *Separate purchase*

CLINICAL SKILLS MANUAL

- *Separate purchase*

 PEARSON eTEXT

- Students can search, highlight, take notes, and more all in electronic format
- *Separate purchase*

 TESTBANK

CHAPTER 39
FAMILY ASSESSMENT AND CONCEPTS OF NURSING CARE IN THE COMMUNITY

LEARNING OUTCOME 1

Categorize the family strengths that help families cope with stressors.

Concepts for Lecture

1. All families experience stressors, which can be positive or negative.
2. Family strengths are the relationships and processes that support and protect families during times of adversity and change.

PowerPoint Slides 26–34

SUGGESTION FOR CLASSROOM ACTIVITIES

- Ask students whether they consider their own families to be "resilient." Why or why not?

SUGGESTION FOR CLINICAL ACTIVITIES

- Families in the hospital setting are often facing stressors. What strategies can the nurse use in the clinical setting to help families cope with these stressors and encourage resilience?

LEARNING OUTCOME 2

Describe the advantages of using a family assessment tool.

Concepts for Lecture

1. Family assessment tools can be used to collect important information about family functioning, coping strategies, family strengths, problem solving, and communication. There are several family assessment tools available.

PowerPoint Slides 35–37

SUGGESTION FOR CLASSROOM ACTIVITIES

- After discussing the available family assessment tools, have students discuss the pros and cons of each tool. What setting is most appropriate for each tool? What information does each tool provide the nurse?

SUGGESTION FOR CLINICAL ACTIVITIES

- Assign students to complete a family assessment using one of the tools discussed in the book. This assessment could occur during clinical care of a hospitalized family, or it could occur in an outpatient or community setting.

LEARNING OUTCOME 3

Identify a variety of family support services that might be available in a community.

Concepts for Lecture

1. Family support services exist in all communities with a purpose of supporting families in the rearing of healthy children. Specific examples of these support services are listed in the PowerPoint slide.

PowerPoint Slides 38–39

SUGGESTION FOR CLASSROOM ACTIVITIES

- Before class, assign students to search the Internet for support services that are available to families in your community. Discuss these services during class.

SUGGESTION FOR CLINICAL ACTIVITIES

- Assign students to attend a program that offers support services for families in your community. Have the student write a reflective journal about the experience.

LEARNING OUTCOME 4

List the variety of community healthcare settings where nurses provide health services to children.

Concepts for Lecture

1. Children receive most of their health care in community settings, and there continues to be a shift to care for children outside of the hospital setting.

LEARNING OUTCOME 5

Describe the role of the nurse in each identified healthcare setting.

Concepts for Lecture

1. Nurses working in the office or healthcare center setting coordinate the health care needed by the child with all other healthcare settings.
2. Nurses working in the school setting focus on promoting health and safety and providing direct care to ill and injured children.
3. Nurses working in childcare settings often serve as consultants in the development of policies. They also train staff and monitor health practices in the setting.
4. Nurses working in the home health setting often care for (or assist families who care for) medically fragile children. They also assess the home environment and assist families in planning for emergencies.

LEARNING OUTCOME 6

Identify emergency care planning that is important in each community setting.

Concepts for Lecture

1. There are many aspects to emergency care planning that can be incorporated into various settings in the community.

  POWERPOINT SLIDES 40–42

 SUGGESTION FOR CLASSROOM ACTIVITIES

- Discuss potential pros and cons of the shift in caring for children in the community rather than in the hospital.

 SUGGESTION FOR CLINICAL ACTIVITIES

- Identify local settings where children potentially receive health care. Determine if RNs provide that care (for example, are there RNs in every school in your community, or do RNs supervise several schools?).

 POWERPOINT SLIDES 43–47

 SUGGESTION FOR CLASSROOM ACTIVITIES

- Use the Weblink Application activity available on *mynursingkit.com* to augment the discussion of this outcome.

 SUGGESTION FOR CLINICAL ACTIVITIES

- Arrange for students to rotate through some of the community settings described in this outcome as part of their clinical rotation.

 POWERPOINT SLIDES 48–52

 VIDEO CLIPS

Emergency: Disaster Preparedness

 VIDEO CLIPS

Emergency: Emergency Medical Services for Children

SUGGESTION FOR CLASSROOM ACTIVITIES

- In many recent disasters, infants and young children have been separated from their families. Discuss strategies that nurses can use to prevent this from happening.

- Explore the possibility of students signing up as volunteers with the local chapter of the Red Cross and completing basic disaster training. In the event of an actual local disaster, students would then be able to directly provide care to those affected.

GENERAL CHAPTER CONSIDERATIONS

1. Have students study and learn key terms listed at beginning of chapter.
2. Have students complete end-of-chapter exercises either in their book or on the MyNursingKit website.
3. Use the Classroom Response Questions provided in PowerPoint to assess students prior to lecture.

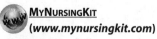
MYNURSINGKIT
(*www.mynursingkit.com*)

- NCLEX RN® review questions
- Case Studies
- Care Plans
- Critical Concept Review
- Thinking Critically
- Weblinks
- Weblink applications
- Nursing Tools
- Audio Glossary
- Images and Tables Library

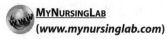
MYNURSINGLAB
(*www.mynursinglab.com*)

- Knowledge Quick Check
- Pre/Posttests
- Customized study plans
- Images and Tables Library
- *Separate purchase*

CLINICAL SKILLS MANUAL

- *Separate purchase*

PEARSON ETEXT

- Students can search, highlight, take notes, and more all in electronic format
- *Separate purchase*

TESTBANK

CHAPTER 40
NURSING CONSIDERATIONS FOR THE CHILD AND FAMILY WITH A CHRONIC CONDITION

LEARNING OUTCOME 1

Discuss causes of chronic conditions in children.

Concepts for Lecture

1. Chronic conditions in children arise from multiple causes, including genetic conditions, congenital defects, insult during birth, and acquired conditions.

POWERPOINT SLIDES 11–12

SUGGESTION FOR CLASSROOM ACTIVITIES

- Write the names of several chronic diseases on index cards. Write the names of the four broad categories of chronic disease discussed in this outcome on the board. Have students place each index card into the correct category.

SUGGESTION FOR CLINICAL ACTIVITIES

- When the students are on a unit, look at the various diagnoses of children being cared for on that unit. Categorize each chronic disease into one of the four broad categories discussed in this outcome.

LEARNING OUTCOME 2

Describe the categories of chronic conditions in children.

Concepts for Lecture

1. Chronic conditions are often defined by diagnostic categories or by functional or social limitations.

POWERPOINT SLIDES 13–15

Table 40–1. Examples of conditions by special healthcare need category

SUGGESTION FOR CLASSROOM ACTIVITIES

- Use the examples listed in Table 40-1: Examples of Conditions by Special Healthcare Need Category to provide examples of diseases in each category discussed in this outcome.

SUGGESTION FOR CLINICAL ACTIVITIES

- Have students talk to a case manager during clinical. Discuss the purpose of categorizing chronic diseases in order to qualify children for special services.

LEARNING OUTCOME 3

Describe the nurse's role in caring for a child with a chronic condition.

Concepts for Lecture

1. The nurse has many roles when caring for a child with a chronic health condition, including providing health supervision, collaboration, referrals, and adaptive parenting behaviors.

LEARNING OUTCOME 4

Assess the family of a child with a chronic condition and discuss the impact of the child's condition on the family.

Concepts for Lecture

1. Assess individual family members' level of understanding of the condition, treatment, and anticipated outcome of the condition.
2. Determine the family's stage of acceptance of the child's chronic illness, and how well the child's care is integrated into family routines.
3. Address the fears and concerns of the family.
4. Provide condition-specific education to help prepare the family for care at home and begin discharge planning.

LEARNING OUTCOME 5

Describe nursing interventions for the child with a chronic condition to support transition to school and adult living.

Concepts for Lecture

1. Nurses can do several things that provide support for families who are transitioning a child with a chronic condition to school or to adult living.

POWERPOINT SLIDES 16–20

SUGGESTION FOR CLASSROOM ACTIVITIES

- Put together a panel of parents who have children with a chronic illness. Ask them to discuss how nurses have played a role in managing their child's illness over time.

SUGGESTION FOR CLINICAL ACTIVITIES

- Place students in outpatient clinics where children with chronic illness are followed. Have students reflect on the role of the nurse in this setting.

POWERPOINT SLIDES 21–26

SUGGESTION FOR CLASSROOM ACTIVITIES

- Before class, assign students to review the Weblink Application "Assisting Parents in Case Management." Use this activity as a basis for discussion during class.

SUGGESTION FOR CLINICAL ACTIVITIES

- Assign students to perform a family assessment of a family caring for a child with a chronic illness. A full discussion of family assessment tools is located in Chapter 39 of the text.

POWERPOINT SLIDES 27–30

SUGGESTION FOR CLASSROOM ACTIVITIES

- Before this class, assign students to complete the activity Case Study, "School Reentry for an Adolescent with a Chronic Condition," on *mynursingkit.com* as a basis for discussion.

SUGGESTION FOR CLINICAL ACTIVITIES

- Identify local resources in the clinical setting that can be used to help families transition to school or to adult living.

LEARNING OUTCOME 6

Discuss the family's role in care coordination.

Concepts for Lecture

1. Families play a major role in coordinating the care of children with chronic illnesses, including determining responsibility for who cares for the child and increased financial expenses. Over time, the family becomes the expert caregivers for their child.

GENERAL CHAPTER CONSIDERATIONS

1. Have students study and learn key terms listed at beginning of chapter.
2. Have students complete end-of-chapter exercises either in their book or on the MyNursingKit website.
3. Use the Classroom Response Questions provided in PowerPoint to assess students prior to lecture.

 POWERPOINT SLIDES 31–33

 SUGGESTION FOR CLASSROOM ACTIVITIES

- Invite a family who cares for a child with a chronic illness in the home setting to speak to your class about their experiences.

 SUGGESTION FOR CLINICAL ACTIVITIES

- When caring for a family who has a child with a chronic illness, encourage the student to explore how the family copes with the child's care in the home setting. Also, the student should assess the possible need for respite care.

 MYNURSINGKIT
(www.mynursingkit.com)

- NCLEX RN® review questions
- Case Studies
- Care Plans
- Critical Concept Review
- Thinking Critically
- Weblinks
- Weblink applications
- Nursing Tools
- Audio Glossary
- Images and Tables Library

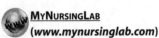 **MYNURSINGLAB**
(www.mynursinglab.com)

- Knowledge Quick Check
- Pre/Posttests
- Customized study plans
- Images and Tables Library
- *Separate purchase*

CLINICAL SKILLS MANUAL

- *Separate purchase*

 PEARSON eTEXT

- Students can search, highlight, take notes, and more all in electronic format
- *Separate purchase*

 TESTBANK

CHAPTER 41
NURSING CONSIDERATIONS FOR THE HOSPITALIZED CHILD

LEARNING OUTCOME 1

Discuss the child's understanding of health and illness according to the child's psychosocial and developmental level.

Concepts for Lecture

1. Children have a different understanding of health and illness than adults. The child's understanding of illness and hospitalization is based primarily on the cognitive ability at different developmental stages and on previous experiences with healthcare professionals.
2. The nurse can classify a child's expected understanding of health and illness based on his or her age.

 POWERPOINT SLIDES 20–27

 SUGGESTION FOR CLASSROOM ACTIVITIES

- Divide the class into four groups, one for each developmental level of the child. Based on their knowledge of how children understand health and illness, have each group identify three techniques the nurse could use when caring for the child in the hospital. Have each group share their ideas with the class.

 SUGGESTION FOR CLINICAL ACTIVITIES

- Suggest that students make small index cards for each developmental group (infants, toddlers, etc.) on which they list the expected understanding of health and illness and techniques to use with that group. When they care for a child, they have a ready reference in their pocket that helps them incorporate developmentally appropriate interventions into their nursing care.

LEARNING OUTCOME 2

Recognize the effect of hospitalization on the child and family.

Concepts for Lecture

1. Hospitalization disrupts a family's usual routines. Parental roles may be altered, and family members may be anxious or fearful.
2. The siblings of a hospitalized child may receive less attention than usual and may feel anxious, guilty, or jealous. See "Teaching Highlights: Strategies for Working with the Sibling of a Hospitalized Child" for details.

 POWERPOINT SLIDES 28–31

 VIDEO CLIPS

Treatment Room

 SUGGESTION FOR CLASSROOM ACTIVITIES

- Invite a panel of parents whose children have been hospitalized to speak to the class. Ask the parents to discuss how the child's hospitalization affected their family, and what nursing interventions were helpful in that situation.

 SUGGESTION FOR CLINICAL ACTIVITIES

- Invite a child life specialist to clinical conference to discuss strategies to help siblings cope with hospitalization.

LEARNING OUTCOME 3

Identify methods that the child and family use to adapt to hospitalization.

Concepts for Lecture

1. Methods that are used to help the child and family adapt to planned hospitalization include tours, therapeutic play, health fairs, and books.
2. During unplanned admissions, the child and family should be oriented to the environment and receive an explanation of procedures.
3. Child life programs can help children and families adapt to hospitalization by providing age-appropriate play, support, and preparation for procedures.

LEARNING OUTCOME 4

Apply family-centered care principles to the hospital setting.

Concepts for Lecture

1. The practice of rooming-in involves a parent staying in the child's hospital room during the course of the child's hospitalization.
2. It is important to continue to promote a child's normal development and usual routines during hospitalization.
3. The nurse can promote family-centered care by orienting families and children to special units and helping them understand what to expect on those units.

LEARNING OUTCOME 5

Identify nursing strategies to minimize the stressors related to hospitalization.

Concepts for Lecture

1. The stress of illness and hospitalization increases the value of play. Specific play activities are based upon the child's level of development. It may be helpful to refer to Table 41–10.
2. Other strategies to minimize the stressors of hospitalization include promoting parental involvement and encouraging parents to support their child.

POWERPOINT SLIDES 32–38

SUGGESTION FOR CLASSROOM ACTIVITIES

- When discussing child life programs, review the Weblink Applications on *mynursingkit.com* to inform the discussion.

SUGGESTION FOR CLINICAL ACTIVITIES

- During orientation to the clinical setting, review which strategies are used in the local clinical facility to promote adaptation to hospitalization

POWERPOINT SLIDES 39–42

SUGGESTION FOR CLASSROOM ACTIVITIES

- Use the activity in the text, "Thinking Critically 41-1: Preparing Children for Hospitalization or Short-Stay Surgery" as a basis for discussing this outcome.

SUGGESTION FOR CLINICAL ACTIVITIES

- When students rotate to specialty units, have them discuss examples of how the unit promotes family-centered care.

POWERPOINT SLIDES 43–50

Table 41–10. Therapeutic play techniques

SUGGESTION FOR CLASSROOM ACTIVITIES

- Bring examples of hospital equipment to the lecture and discuss which types of equipment are safe for children to play with and which ones are not.

SUGGESTION FOR CLINICAL ACTIVITIES

- Role model age-appropriate play for students using toys found in the clinical setting.

LEARNING OUTCOME 6

Discuss family presence during procedures and nursing strategies used to prepare the family.

Concepts for Lecture

1. Most parents want to be present during procedures in order to support their child and to know what is happening during the procedure. The nurse can discuss the extent to which parents want to be involved in order to prepare them for the procedure.

PowerPoint Slides 51–52

Suggestion for Classroom Activities

• Ask students to imagine that they are parents who have a child undergoing venipuncture in a treatment room. The child is crying. Which would be more stressful for the parent: Seeing what is happening or imagining what is happening through a closed door? Point out that many children cry due to separation from parents or during restraint.

Suggestion for Clinical Activities

• Point out the treatment room that is used for procedures and discuss the unit's practice regarding parental presence during procedures.

LEARNING OUTCOME 7

Discuss strategies for preparing children and families for discharge from the hospital setting

Concepts for Lecture

1. Nurses help to coordinate the multidisciplinary team in order to prepare children for discharge.
2. The nurse assesses the family's ability to manage a child's care at home. This process begins upon admission to the hospital.
3. The nurse teaches the family special skills that are needed to care for the child at home.

PowerPoint Slides 53–56

Suggestion for Classroom Activities

• Use the activity in the textbook "Critical Thinking in Action" as a framework for discussion about the nurse's role in discharge teaching.

Suggestion for Clinical Activities

• Assign students to spend part of a clinical day with a case coordinator who is responsible for discharge planning. Have students write a reflective journal of this experience.

GENERAL CHAPTER CONSIDERATIONS

1. Have students study and learn key terms listed at beginning of chapter.
2. Have students complete end-of-chapter exercises either in their book or on the MyNursingKit website.
3. Use the Classroom Response Questions provided in PowerPoint to assess students prior to lecture.

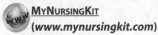

MyNursingKit
(*www.mynursingkit.com*)

- NCLEX RN® review questions
- Case Studies
- Care Plans
- Critical Concept Review
- Thinking Critically
- Weblinks
- Weblink applications
- Nursing Tools
- Audio Glossary
- Images and Tables Library

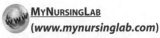

MyNursingLab
(*www.mynursinglab.com*)

- Knowledge Quick Check
- Pre/Posttests
- Customized study plans
- Images and Tables Library
- *Separate purchase*

CLINICAL SKILLS MANUAL

- *Separate purchase*

PEARSON eTEXT

- Students can search, highlight, take notes, and more all in electronic format
- *Separate purchase*

TESTBANK

CHAPTER 42
PAIN ASSESSMENT
AND MANAGEMENT IN CHILDREN

LEARNING OUTCOME 1

Identify the physiologic and behavioral consequences of pain in infants and children.

Concepts for Lecture

1. Many beliefs about children and pain are outdated. We now know that neonates do feel pain, infants can remember pain, parents rarely exaggerate their child's pain, and that children rarely get addicted to pain medication. Although children heal from surgery faster than adults, they still experience the same amount of pain. See Table 42–1 for details.
2. The clinical manifestations of pain can be seen both physiologically and behaviorally.
3. Short-term consequences of pain include respiratory changes, neurological changes, metabolic changes, immune system changes, gastrointestinal changes, and increased pain sensitivity. Long-term consequences of pain are not well-known.

POWERPOINT SLIDES 16–23

Figure 42–4. Neonatal pain facial expression

Table 42–1. Misconceptions about pain in infants and children

Table 42–3. Physiologic consequences of unrelieved pain in children

VIDEO CLIPS

Pain Perception

SUGGESTION FOR CLASSROOM ACTIVITIES

- Ask students to think back to their own childhood. Can they recall a time when they had severe pain? What was the cause? How was it treated? Do they believe that it affected them?

SUGGESTION FOR CLINICAL ACTIVITIES

- During the clinical day, find an infant whom the students can examine. Have them state what physiologic and behavioral indicators they would look for to determine if the child is experiencing pain.

LEARNING OUTCOME 2

Assess the developmental abilities of children to perform a self-assessment of pain intensity.

Concepts for Lecture

1. There are numerous tools available to assess pain in infants and children. The appropriate tool varies by age.
2. An appropriate tool for measuring pain in neonates is the Neonatal Infant Pain Scale (NIPS). See Table 42–4.
3. For infants, the NIPS or the FLACC Behavioral Pain Assessment Scale may be used. See Tables 42–4 and 42–5.
4. Toddlers may be able to self-report pain, but they cannot be given more than three choices on a pain scale (such as none, some, a lot).

POWERPOINT SLIDES 24–30

Table 42–4. Neonatal infant pain scale (NIPS)

Table 42–5. FLACC behavioral pain assessment scale

SUGGESTION FOR CLASSROOM ACTIVITIES

- During the discussion on pain scales, go to the Oucher Scale Website (see weblinks on *mynursingkit.com; www.oucher.org*). Briefly discuss the importance of using a tool that has been tested for reliability and validity. Ask students why it is important for the Oucher Scale to be available for multiple ethnicities.

5. Once children can understand rank and order, they can use a numerical scale to report pain. Examples of self-report pain scales include the Faces Pain Rating Scale and the Oucher Scale.
6. By about the age of 8, children can also describe pain in more detail (such as sharp, dull, aching, etc.).

LEARNING OUTCOME 3

Describe the nursing assessment and management for a child receiving an opioid analgesic.

Concepts for Lecture

1. Opioid analgesics are commonly given for severe pain, such as after surgery or a severe injury. They may be administered by the oral, subcutaneous, intramuscular, rectal, and intravenous routes, although the oral and intravenous routes are preferred for children.
2. Dosage of analgesics in children is always weight-based. Refer to the *Drug Guide for Opioid Analgesics and Recommended Doses for Children and Adolescents*. Common side effects of opioids include sedation, nausea, vomiting, constipation, and itching. Less common complications include respiratory depression, cardiovascular collapse, and addiction. Knowing the time of peak drug effect can help the nurse monitor for serious side effects. Naloxone (Narcan) should be available to treat respiratory depression.
3. Pain relief should be provided around the clock, as delays in giving analgesics increase the chances of breakthrough pain. Patient-controlled analgesia (PCA) may be used with children, especially in the first 48 hours after surgery.
4. Withdrawal may occur when opioids have been given for an extended period of time. See Table 42–6 for signs and symptoms of withdrawal.
5. Other drugs are used as adjuncts to pain management in children and are dosed by weight.

LEARNING OUTCOME 4

Explain the physiology that enables nonpharmacologic (complementary) methods of pain control to be effective.

Concepts for Lecture

1. The Gate Control Theory helps explain why complementary pain management techniques are effective in helping to control pain. Refer to "Pathophysiology Illustrated: Pain Perception" when discussing this theory.
2. Methods of nonpharmacologic interventions include distraction cutaneous stimulation, sucrose solution, electroanalgesia, guided imagery, relaxation, hypnosis, acupuncture, and heat or cold application.

SUGGESTION FOR CLINICAL ACTIVITIES
• Have students review "Skill 13–1: Selected Pediatric Pain Scales," from the *Clinical Skills Manual* before attending clinical conference.

REFERENCE
www.oucher.org

POWERPOINT SLIDES 31–40

Table 42–6. Clinical manifestations of opioid or sedative withdrawal

ANIMATION
Morphine

VIDEO CLIPS
Pain Management Kit

SUGGESTIONS FOR CLASSROOM ACTIVITIES
• When discussing opioids, show the animation "Morphine," from *mynursingkit.com*. The animation provides a visual about how opioids act to treat pain.
• Show the video "Pain Management Kit."
• Before discussing patient-controlled analgesia, review "Skill 13–2: Patient-Controlled Analgesia," from the Clinical Skills Manual.

SUGGESTION FOR CLINICAL ACTIVITIES
• Role play with students about what they would do if a child receiving opioids suffered from respiratory depression. What equipment and medications would they need? What actions would be the first priority?

POWERPOINT SLIDES 41–44

SUGGESTION FOR CLASSROOM ACTIVITIES
• Have students read "Complementary Care: Complementary Therapies for Pain Control." Ask students if they have ever seen hypnosis used in the hospital setting. If a parent requested this option, what could the nurse do to advocate for hypnotherapy?

SUGGESTION FOR CLINICAL ACTIVITIES

- During clinical conference, have students discuss how parents can help children cope with pain. Interventions vary by age. "Teaching Highlights: Helping a Child Cope with Pain" is a good reference for this discussion.

LEARNING OUTCOME 5

Assess children of different ages with acute pain and develop a nursing care plan that integrates pharmacologic interventions and developmentally appropriate nonpharmacologic (complementary) therapies.

Concepts for Lecture

1. The nursing process can be applied as a framework for working with children of all ages who are experiencing acute pain. "Nursing Care Plan: The Child with Postoperative Pain" is a good reference for this discussion.
2. Interventions are most effective when age considerations are taken into account.

POWERPOINT SLIDES 45–54

SUGGESTION FOR CLASSROOM ACTIVITIES

- Approach this care plan using a case study format. Suggestions may be found on *mynursingkit.com* in the Weblink Applications. This approach helps students apply the nursing process to a realistic case.

SUGGESTION FOR CLINICAL ACTIVITIES

- Before clinical conference, have students complete the "Case Study: Postoperative Pain Assessment" activity, from the Companion Website at *mynursingkit.com*. Compare their answers to the process or protocol used in the actual hospital. If there is no written protocol or order set in place, discuss the benefits of such a protocol for making care more consistent and increasing nursing autonomy.

LEARNING OUTCOME 6

Develop a nursing care plan for assessing and monitoring the child having sedation and analgesia for a medical procedure.

Concepts for Lecture

1. Pain control should be provided for children undergoing both major and minor procedures. The anticipation of the procedure can be very anxiety-provoking for the child, and poor pain control during prior procedures can lead to a very uncooperative child.
2. Topical anesthetics can be used to prevent pain for minor procedures such as venipuncture and IV starts.
3. Sedation is used during major medical procedures, with the goal being to provide both analgesia and anxiolysis.
4. Nursing responsibilities for the child receiving sedation involves considerations about timing of drug administration, as well as monitoring during the procedure.

POWERPOINT SLIDES 55–66

Figure 42–6. Technique for applying EMLA cream

Table 42–7. Characteristics of minimal, moderate, and deep sedation

VIDEO CLIPS

Nursing in Action: Conscious Sedation Monitoring

SUGGESTION FOR CLASSROOM ACTIVITIES

- Before students come to class, assign them to review "Skill 13-3: Monitoring Sedation" from the *Clinical Skills Manual*. Use this skill as a basis for discussion.

SUGGESTION FOR CLINICAL ACTIVITIES

- Discuss the concept of "thinking ahead." For example, if a child is receiving light sedation, what equipment should be available in the event that the child progresses into deep sedation? What interventions should occur? What medications would be administered? By thinking through these potential problems before they occur, students can be better prepared to deal with them if they actually occur.

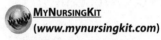 **MYNURSINGKIT**
(*www.mynursingkit.com*)

- NCLEX RN® review questions
- Case Studies
- Care Plans
- Critical Concept Review
- Thinking Critically
- Weblinks
- Weblink applications
- Nursing Tools
- Audio Glossary
- Images and Tables Library

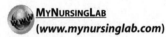 **MYNURSINGLAB**
(*www.mynursinglab.com*)

- Knowledge Quick Check
- Pre/Posttests
- Customized study plans
- Images and Tables Library
- *Separate purchase*

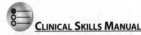 **CLINICAL SKILLS MANUAL**

- *Separate purchase*

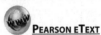 **PEARSON ETEXT**

- Students can search, highlight, take notes, and more all in electronic format
- *Separate purchase*

 TESTBANK

GENERAL CHAPTER CONSIDERATIONS

1. Have students study and learn key terms listed at beginning of chapter.
2. Have students complete end-of-chapter exercises either in their book or on the MyNursingKit website.
3. Use the Classroom Response Questions provided in PowerPoint to assess students prior to lecture.

CHAPTER 43
THE CHILD WITH A LIFE-THREATENING CONDITION AND END-OF-LIFE CARE

LEARNING OUTCOME 1

Describe the child's experiences with life-threatening illness or injury according to developmental level.

Concepts for Lecture

1. Because children of various ages are at different stages of development, their responses to illness and injury vary. Table 41-1 (in Chapter 41) summarizes this information.

POWERPOINT SLIDES 20–30

Table 41–1. (from Chapter 41) Stressors of hospitalization for children at various developmental stages

SUGGESTION FOR CLASSROOM ACTIVITIES

- Discuss nursing interventions that can be used to address children's responses to hospitalization based on developmental levels. Refer to Table 41-1 for suggestions.

SUGGESTION FOR CLINICAL ACTIVITIES

- Invite a member of the child life staff to speak with students at a clinical conference about children's responses to hospitalization and illness.

LEARNING OUTCOME 2

Discuss the family's experience and reactions to having a child with a life-threatening illness or injury.

Concepts for Lecture

1. Parents typically respond to a life-threatening illness in their child by displaying emotions such as shock, disbelief, anger, and guilt. Table 43-1 is a good reference.
2. Siblings of a critically ill child often may feel resentment or anger toward the ill child. Normal family routines are altered, and the siblings may feel ignored and forgotten.

POWERPOINT SLIDES 31–38

Table 43–1. Nursing interventions to meet parental needs when the child is hospitalized with a life-threatening illness or injury

VIDEO CLIPS

Involving Family in NICU Setting

SUGGESTIONS FOR CLASSROOM ACTIVITIES

- Show the video "Involving Family in NICU Setting," available on *mynurskingkit.com* Ask the class how the nursing staff can involve the family in the critical-care setting.
- Clip out various obituaries from the local paper from children who have died. Based on the message and tone, have the students identify what stage of grief the family was in when they wrote the obituary.

- Identify resources available that the bedside nurse in the local clinical setting can use to help support families and siblings during times of stress. Examples include social workers, chaplains, child life specialists, case managers, therapists, and advanced practice nurses.

POWERPOINT SLIDES 39–43

LEARNING OUTCOME 3

Describe the coping mechanisms used by the child and family in response to stress.

Concepts for Lecture

1. Children and adults use various methods to cope with illness and injury within the family.

SUGGESTION FOR CLASSROOM ACTIVITIES

- Ask students to share examples of the coping mechanisms discussed in this outcome.

SUGGESTION FOR CLINICAL ACTIVITIES

- When caring for hospitalized children, remind students to be alert for coping mechanisms that children may be using. Discuss ways the nurse can allow the child to use these coping mechanisms.

LEARNING OUTCOME 4

Develop a nursing care plan for the child with a life-threatening illness or injury.

Concepts for Lecture

1. The nursing care of the child with a life-threatening illness or injury includes reducing anxiety, relieving powerlessness, and treating pain. "Nursing Care Plan: The Child Coping with a Life-Threatening Illness or Injury" provides details about these interventions.

POWERPOINT SLIDES 44–48

SUGGESTION FOR CLASSROOM ACTIVITIES

- Discuss how nurses can help children maintain routines while the child is hospitalized.

SUGGESTION FOR CLINICAL ACTIVITIES

- Identify pain scales that are used in the local clinical setting to assess pain in children of various ages.

LEARNING OUTCOME 5

Apply assessment skills to identify the physiologic changes that occur in the dying child.

Concepts for Lecture

1. The human body goes through many physiologic changes as it dies. "Clinical Manifestations: The Dying Child" reviews these changes in detail.

POWERPOINT SLIDES 49–56

Table 43–3. Strategies for communicating with the dying child

SUGGESTION FOR CLASSROOM ACTIVITIES

- As you discuss the clinical manifestations of death, discuss common interventions used to promote comfort during death. For example, air hunger may be treated with opioids, head of bed elevation, and increased airflow in the room.

SUGGESTION FOR CLINICAL ACTIVITIES

- Have students role-play how they would talk to a dying child. Refer to Table 43-3 for specific strategies.

LEARNING OUTCOME 6

Develop a nursing care plan to provide family-centered care for the dying child and the family.

Concepts for Lecture

1. Nursing interventions appropriate for the family with a dying child include providing physical comfort for the child, providing emotional comfort, maintaining family functioning, and promoting cultural values. Table 43-4 and Table 43-5 are helpful references.

 POWERPOINT SLIDES 57–60

Table 43–4. Cultural traditions in mourning and after-death rites

Table 43–5. Children's understanding of death and possible behavioral responses

VIDEO CLIPS

Presenting Bad News to Families

VIDEO CLIPS

Parental Reactions to Death of a Child

SUGGESTIONS FOR CLASSROOM ACTIVITIES

There are numerous resources that can be used to augment this outcome:

* Videos on *mynursingkit.com:* "Presenting Bad News to Families" and "Parental Reactions to Death of a Child."
* *mynursingkit.com* activity: "Critical Thinking in Action: Helping the Family Cope with the Death of a Premature Infant."
* Discuss "Complementary Care: Prayer" in the textbook.

SUGGESTION FOR CLINICAL ACTIVITIES

* If there is a local support group for bereaved parents, arrange for students to observe a meeting.

LEARNING OUTCOME 7

Implement strategies for bereavement support of the parents and siblings after the death of a child.

Concepts for Lecture

1. Nurses can provide support to both parents and siblings after the death of a child. These interventions help the family during the grieving process.

 POWERPOINT SLIDES 61–63

SUGGESTION FOR CLASSROOM ACTIVITIES

* Before class, have students search the Internet for resources that are available to support grieving families and siblings in your local area. Discuss these resources during class.

SUGGESTION FOR CLINICAL ACTIVITIES

* Have students identify resources in the clinical setting that may be used to support children and families nearing death. These materials may include written materials, art materials, handprints or footprints, and so on.

LEARNING OUTCOME 8

Describe strategies to support nurses who care for children who die.

Concepts for Lecture

1. Caring for dying children is very stressful, and it is natural for nurses to feel a sense of loss and grief when a child dies.
2. Support systems and debriefing groups are helpful resources for nurses who care for dying children.

GENERAL CHAPTER CONSIDERATIONS

1. Have students study and learn key terms listed at beginning of chapter.
2. Have students complete end-of-chapter exercises either in their book or on the MyNursingKit website.
3. Use the Classroom Response Questions provided in PowerPoint to assess students prior to lecture.

 POWERPOINT SLIDES 64–68

Figure 43–7. Nurses' need for support

 SUGGESTION FOR CLASSROOM ACTIVITIES

- Invite a panel of pediatric nurses to attend class and discuss how they cope with the death of children that they care for. This panel works best when there is a wide range of nurses represented: men, women, critical care nurses, acute care nurses, and so on. Have the students prepare one or two questions in advance to ask the panel.

 SUGGESTION FOR CLINICAL ACTIVITIES

- Many hospitals have formal support programs for staff when a child dies. If such a program exists in your clinical setting, arrange for the facilitator to come to a clinical conference to discuss self-care actions that nurses can use when children they are caring for die.

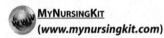 **MYNURSINGKIT**
(www.mynursingkit.com)

- NCLEX RN® review questions
- Case Studies
- Care Plans
- Critical Concept Review
- Thinking Critically
- Weblinks
- Weblink applications
- Nursing Tools
- Audio Glossary
- Images and Tables Library

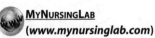 **MYNURSINGLAB**
(www.mynursinglab.com)

- Knowledge Quick Check
- Pre/Posttests
- Customized study plans
- Images and Tables Library
- *Separate purchase*

CLINICAL SKILLS MANUAL

- *Separate purchase*

 PEARSON ETEXT

- Students can search, highlight, take notes, and more all in electronic format
- *Separate purchase*

 TESTBANK

CHAPTER 44
SOCIAL AND ENVIRONMENTAL INFLUENCES ON THE CHILD

LEARNING OUTCOME 1

Identify major social and environmental factors that influence the health of children and adolescents.

Concepts for Lecture

1. Many social and environmental factors influence children's health. Most morbidity is related to preventable causes, such as car crashes, fires, drowning, and homicides. Mental disorders and pregnancy are common reasons for adolescents to be admitted to the hospital.

 POWERPOINT SLIDES 22–25

 SUGGESTION FOR CLASSROOM ACTIVITIES

- Assign students to develop parent or child teaching plans focused on stress management for children of various ages. Compare stress risks and strategies for different age groups.

 SUGGESTION FOR CLINICAL ACTIVITIES

- Determine the causes of death for children in the local community. Do they coincide with national statistics? What social and environmental factors do local experts believe have the greatest impact on children's health?

LEARNING OUTCOME 2

List external influences that influence child and adolescent health.

Concepts for Lecture

1. External influences that affect child and adolescent health include poverty, stress, family structure, school and child care, community, and culture.

 POWERPOINT SLIDES 26–37

 SUGGESTION FOR CLASSROOM ACTIVITIES

- During class, have students read "Evidence-Based Nursing: Homelessness from the Viewpoint of Mothers and Children," located in the main textbook. Incorporate the findings from this study into the discussion about homelessness.

 SUGGESTION FOR CLINICAL ACTIVITIES

- Students will likely care for children and families who are homeless or live in poverty. Have students identify local community resources to which they can refer families.

LEARNING OUTCOME 3

Apply the ecological model and resilience theory to assessment of the social and environmental factors in children's lives.

 POWERPOINT SLIDES 38–42

 SUGGESTION FOR CLASSROOM ACTIVITIES

- Create a list of protective factors and risk factors and list them in random order on the board. Have the students identify which factors are protective and which ones are risk factors as you discuss resiliency theory.

Concepts for Lecture

1. The ecological model views the child and the environment as interacting forces. Children influence the systems around them, and the systems in turn influence the child.
2. Resilience theory examines risk and protective factors in the child's environment.

LEARNING OUTCOME 4

Examine the effects of substance use, physical activity, and other lifestyle patterns on health.

Concepts for Lecture

1. Tobacco use is the most preventable cause of adult death in the United States. Most adults begin smoking during their teenage years.
2. Substance abuse occurs in children and adolescents of all socioeconomic levels and is a growing health problem.
3. Physical inactivity reflects our society's lifestyle. Children have become increasingly sedentary, which has led to a rise in childhood obesity.
4. Other lifestyle patterns that can influence the health of children and adolescents include the use of protective equipment, body art, and sexual orientation.

SUGGESTION FOR CLINICAL ACTIVITIES

- When students are completing care plans for children and families they have cared for, have them incorporate the ecological model or resiliency theory into their care plan. This encourages students to consider the effect of various systems on the child's health status.

POWERPOINT SLIDES 43–59

Figure 44–5. Role of sports in development

Figure 44–6. Use of protective gear

VIDEO CLIPS

Identifying Youth Who Abuse Drugs and Alcohol Use

VIDEO CLIPS

Smoking and Smoking Cessation

VIDEO CLIPS

Extreme Sports

SUGGESTIONS FOR CLASSROOM ACTIVITIES

- In class, view the videos on "Smoking and Smoking Cessation" and "Identifying Youth Who Abuse Drugs and Alcohol Use" available on *mynursingkit.com*. Invite a substance abuse counselor to class to discuss adolescent patterns of drug and alcohol use and abuse.
- Watch the video "Extreme Sports" available on *mynursingkit.com* and assign "Weblink Applications: Develop a Teaching Plan: Individualized Sport" activity for students to complete in-class. Allow time to discuss answers.

SUGGESTION FOR CLINICAL ACTIVITIES

- Role play with students how they might approach a teenager who is engaging in one or more of the behaviors discussed in this outcome.

LEARNING OUTCOME 5

Plan nursing interventions for children who experience violence.

Concepts for Lecture

1. Potential sources of violence involving children include violence in the media, abuse, homicide, terrorist attacks, and wars.
2. There are many nursing interventions that can be applied to children experiencing violence. Tables 44-5 and 44-6 are helpful references.

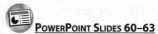
PowerPoint Slides 60–63

Table 44-5. Risk factors common in families with child victims of violence

Table 44-6. Assessment questions to identify violence risk and protective factors

Video Clips

Violence in the Media

Suggestion for Classroom Activities

- During class, show the video "Violence in the Media," available on *mynursingkit.com*. Use this as a basis for the discussion about violence.

Suggestion for Clinical Activities

- Ask students to pay attention to the types of TV shows, movies, and computer games that children watch and play in the hospital setting. Many times these activities contain excessive violence, which provides the nurse an opportunity to address the issue with the child and family.

LEARNING OUTCOME 6

Evaluate the environment for hazards to children, such as exposure to substances and potential for poisoning.

Concepts for Lecture

1. Poisoning is a common occurrence in pediatrics, and most poisonings occur in the home. Young children, ages 1 to 4, are at the highest risk for poisoning. Prevention of poisoning by assessing the home for potentially toxic substances is important.
2. Foreign objects are most likely to be ingested by children who are 6 months to 3 years of age. Common objects ingested include coins, pins, toys, batteries, and bones from food.
3. The removal of lead from paint has significantly decreased the incidence of lead poisoning; however, children who live in older houses remain at risk for lead poisoning.

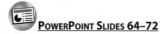
PowerPoint Slides 64–72

Animation

Activated Charcoal

Animation

Lead Poisoning

Suggestion for Classroom Activities

- Play "Guess the Toxin" using the Clinical Manifestations: Commonly Ingested Toxic Agents feature in this chapter. Have groups of students create a brief case study of a child with toxin ingestion. Use the clinical manifestations as a potential symptom list. Have the groups present their case to the class and see if the class can figure out what toxin caused the symptoms.

Suggestion for Clinical Activities

- Discuss the treatment of poisonings in the emergency department and the role of antidotes, lavage, activated charcoal, and cathartics.

LEARNING OUTCOME 7

Explore the nursing role in prevention and treatment of child abuse and neglect, and other forms of violence.

Concepts for Lecture

1. Abuse is a relatively common form of violence inflicted on children, and can involve neglect, physical abuse, emotional abuse, or sexual abuse. The most common perpetrator of abuse is the parent or guardian of the child. There are numerous risk factors that are associated with abusive behavior.
2. Prevention and treatment of abuse center on promotion of parenting skills, detection of abuse, and reporting.

 POWERPOINT SLIDES 73–78

 VIDEO CLIPS

Identifying Child Abuse

 SUGGESTION FOR CLASSROOM ACTIVITIES

- During the discussion of this outcome, view the video "Identifying Child Abuse," available on the *mynursingkit.com* website.

 SUGGESTION FOR CLINICAL ACTIVITIES

- Invite a social worker from your local child protection services department to talk with the students about detections of child abuse and reporting requirements for nurses.

LEARNING OUTCOME 8

Plan nursing interventions for children related to social and environmental situations.

Concepts for Lecture

1. Many nursing interventions related to social and environmental situations involve teaching health promotion behaviors that emphasize prevention.

 POWERPOINT SLIDES 79–80

 SUGGESTION FOR CLASSROOM ACTIVITIES

- Assign students to locate resources that relate to topics discussed in this outcome (such as teaching materials for families about gun safety, lead exposure, etc.) and use these materials as a framework for discussing this content

 SUGGESTION FOR CLINICAL ACTIVITIES

- Have students identify opportunities during clinical to teach families focused information about one of the topics in this chapter (such as lead exposure, toxin exposure, or gun safety).

GENERAL CHAPTER CONSIDERATIONS

1. Have students study and learn key terms listed at beginning of chapter.
2. Have students complete end-of-chapter exercises either in their book or on the MyNursingKit website.
3. Use the Classroom Response Questions provided in PowerPoint to assess students prior to lecture.

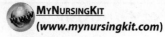

MyNursingKit
(*www.mynursingkit.com*)

- NCLEX RN® review questions
- Case Studies
- Care Plans
- Critical Concept Review
- Thinking Critically
- Weblinks
- Weblink applications
- Nursing Tools
- Audio Glossary
- Images and Tables Library

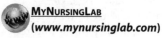

MyNursingLab
(*www.mynursinglab.com*)

- Knowledge Quick Check
- Pre/Posttests
- Customized study plans
- Images and Tables Library
- *Separate purchase*

CLINICAL SKILLS MANUAL

- *Separate purchase*

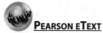

PEARSON eTEXT

- Students can search, highlight, take notes, and more all in electronic format
- *Separate purchase*

TESTBANK

CHAPTER 45
IMMUNIZATION
AND COMMUNICABLE DISEASES

LEARNING OUTCOME 1

Describe the reasons why children are more vulnerable than adults to infectious and communicable diseases.

Concepts for Lecture

1. Infants are particularly vulnerable to diseases for several reasons. Their immune systems are not fully mature at birth. The antibodies that are passively acquired from their mothers have limited protection, and this protection further decreases over time. Finally, infants have incomplete disease protection until they receive immunizations.
2. Children get exposed to diseases through interactions with other children and adults. This exposure to illness allows them to naturally develop antibodies to these diseases, which prevents subsequent infections from the same organism.
3. Many behaviors of children contribute to the ease with which infections are transmitted, including poor hygiene and handwashing.

LEARNING OUTCOME 2

Describe the process of infection and modes of transmission.

Concepts for Lecture

1. An infectious disease is any communicable disease caused by microorganisms that are commonly transmitted from one person to another, or from an animal to a person. A communicable disease is an illness directly or indirectly transmitted from one person or animal to another by contact with body fluids, contaminated items, or by vectors (such as ticks, mosquitoes, etc.).
2. For a communicable disease to occur, three links need to be present: an infectious agent or pathogen, an effective means of transmission, and a susceptible host. The pathogen must also have a suitable reservoir, or habitat, that can be living or nonliving. Transmission may be direct or indirect.
3. Infection control aims to interrupt the chain of transmission, or eliminate either the reservoir or the habitat.

LEARNING OUTCOME 3

Explain the role that vaccines play in reducing and eliminating communicable diseases.

Concepts for Lecture

1. Vaccines introduce an antigen into the body. An antigen is a foreign substance that triggers an immune response, and an antibody is a protein produced by the body in response to the antigen.

 POWERPOINT SLIDES 21–24

 SUGGESTION FOR CLASSROOM ACTIVITIES

- Discuss how the nurse can help children and families learn how to prevent disease transmission. "Teaching Highlights: Reducing the Transmission of Infection" can be used to generate ideas for the discussion.

 SUGGESTION FOR CLINICAL ACTIVITIES

- Hospitalized children often do not wash their hands after toileting or before eating. Discuss the importance of teaching children proper handwashing techniques, as well as how the nurse can teach these techniques during hospitalization.

 POWERPOINT SLIDES 25–29

Feature Box: Pathophysiology Illustrated: The Chain of Infection Transmission

 SUGGESTION FOR CLASSROOM ACTIVITIES

- When discussing the chain of infection, use influenza as an example. Most students have had influenza and can relate the disease to the concepts discussed.

 SUGGESTION FOR CLINICAL ACTIVITIES

- Discuss how infection control methods commonly used in the hospital affect the chain of infection. Specifically, why do different pathogens have different infection control methods (such as contact versus droplet)?

 POWERPOINT SLIDES 30–39

Figure 45–2A. Recommended immunization schedule for children 0 to 6 years, United States, 2008

Figure 45–2B. Recommended immunization schedule for children and adolescents 7 to 18 years, United States, 2008

2. Active immunity occurs when antibody production is stimulated without causing clinical disease. The body must have the ability to make antibodies for immunity to occur. Passive immunity can be induced with antibodies produced in another human or animal host.

3. Many diseases have been nearly eliminated or significantly decreased due to vaccinations. Overall, there are many benefits to vaccination.

4. Types of vaccines used in the United States include killed virus vaccines, toxoids, live virus vaccines, recombinant forms, and conjugated forms.

5. The schedule for vaccination is routinely updated and is available on the CDC website. For the 2008 recommendations, refer to Figure 45-2. Supplemental immunizations for certain children are summarized in Table 45-1.

6. There are numerous barriers to vaccination, including limited access to health care, inadequate education about the importance of vaccination, and religious prohibitions. An increasing number of parents are choosing not to vaccinate their children, which could have a significant impact on the health of their own child and other children in the community.

LEARNING OUTCOME 4

Develop a nursing care plan for children of all ages needing immunizations.

Concepts for Lecture

1. Assessment and diagnosis by the nurse are the first steps in the care of a child needing immunizations. "Nursing Care Plan: The Child Needing Immunizations" is a good reference.

2. Planning involves advocating for immunization, informing parents about side effects, and obtaining consent.

3. Implementation includes administration of the vaccine, as well as documentation. Adverse events must be reported by law—refer to Table 45-2.

4. Evaluation serves as a way for the nurse to verify that nursing care was complete and thorough.

LEARNING OUTCOME 5

Outline a plan to maintain the potency of vaccines.

Concepts for Lecture

1. Vaccines must be stored properly in order to maintain potency. There are several methods that can be used to maintain proper storage requirements.

Table 45-1. Supplemental immunizations

SUGGESTION FOR CLASSROOM ACTIVITIES

- Distribute copies of the latest vaccination schedule to the class (or, have them download their own copy from the CDC website). Using different ages, ask what immunizations the child would receive if he or she presented to the clinic. After the students understand how to interpret the chart, have them determine how to catch a child up on missed vaccines.

SUGGESTION FOR CLINICAL ACTIVITIES

- An 8-year-old child comes in for an appendectomy, and while taking the health history the parent states that the child has never received any immunizations. How might the nurse further explore this issue with the parent?

POWERPOINT SLIDES 40–48

Table 45-2. Common misconceptions about vaccines and correct information

SUGGESTION FOR CLASSROOM ACTIVITIES

- Have students review "Case Study: Indecision over Vaccination," located on *mynursingkit.com*. Use the case study as a stimulus for discussion during this outcome.

SUGGESTION FOR CLINICAL ACTIVITIES

- Children are often extremely fearful of immunizations, and have often had negative experiences with prior immunizations. During clinical conference, discuss how to reduce children's pain and anxiety during immunizations.

POWERPOINT SLIDES 49–51

SUGGESTION FOR CLASSROOM ACTIVITIES

- If vaccines are not stored properly, they should be discarded. Have students research the cost of vaccines before class so that they also understand the financial implications with storing vaccines properly.

SUGGESTION FOR CLINICAL ACTIVITIES

- During clinical, have students locate the storage area for vaccines and determine which processes are in place to maintain the potency of the vaccines.

LEARNING OUTCOME 6

Recognize common infectious and communicable diseases.

Concepts for Lecture

1. Infectious and communicable diseases that may be seen during childhood (summarized in Table 45-4 include chickenpox, coxsackievirus, diphtheria, fifth disease, *Haemophilus influenzae* type B, influenza, measles, mononucleosis, mumps, pertussis, pneumococcus, poliomyelitis, roseola, rotavirus, rubella, streptococcus A, and tetanus.
2. Infectious diseases that are commonly transmitted by insect or animal hosts (summarized in Table 45-5) include Lyme disease, malaria, rabies, and Rocky Mountain Spotted Fever.

LEARNING OUTCOME 7

Develop a nursing care plan for a child with a common communicable disease.

Concepts for Lecture

1. The nursing process can be applied to children with communicable diseases.

POWERPOINT SLIDES 52–100

Table 45–4. Selected infectious and communicable diseases in children

Table 45–5. Selected infectious diseases transmitted by insect or animal hosts (zoonosis)

SUGGESTION FOR CLASSROOM ACTIVITIES

- Before class, divide students into groups and have each group be responsible for briefly presenting each infectious disease discussed in this chapter. Encourage them to locate pictures of the diseases, as the skin patterns are very important in the recognition of the disease.

SUGGESTION FOR CLINICAL ACTIVITIES

- It is difficult to remember the isolation requirements for each of these infectious diseases. Identify resources available in the clinical setting that nurses can refer to for specific information about these diseases.

POWERPOINT SLIDES 101–106

SUGGESTION FOR CLASSROOM ACTIVITIES

- Assign students to complete this outcome before class and bring the care plan with them to class. Have students trade care plans and critique each other's work.

SUGGESTION FOR CLINICAL ACTIVITIES

- During clinical conference, discuss nonpharmacologic strategies for managing fever in children.

GENERAL CHAPTER CONSIDERATIONS

1. Have students study and learn key terms listed at beginning of chapter.
2. Have students complete end-of-chapter exercises either in their book or on the MyNursingKit website.
3. Use the Classroom Response Questions provided in PowerPoint to assess students prior to lecture.

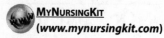

MyNursingKit
(*www.mynursingkit.com*)

- NCLEX RN® review questions
- Case Studies
- Care Plans
- Critical Concept Review
- Thinking Critically
- Weblinks
- Weblink applications
- Nursing Tools
- Audio Glossary
- Images and Tables Library

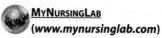

MyNursingLab
(*www.mynursinglab.com*)

- Knowledge Quick Check
- Pre/Posttests
- Customized study plans
- Images and Tables Library
- *Separate purchase*

CLINICAL SKILLS MANUAL

- *Separate purchase*

PEARSON eTEXT

- Students can search, highlight, take notes, and more all in electronic format
- *Separate purchase*

TESTBANK

CHAPTER 46
THE CHILD WITH ALTERATIONS IN FLUID, ELECTROLYTE, AND ACID-BASE BALANCE

LEARNING OUTCOME 1

Describe normal fluid and electrolyte status for children at various ages.

Concepts for Lecture

1. Fluid and electrolytes are highly regulated in the human body. A basic vocabulary is necessary to discuss the location and flow of fluids in the body.
2. Neonates and young infants have a proportionately larger extracellular fluid volume than older children and adults, and they are vulnerable to dehydration.
3. Infants and children under age 2 lose a greater proportion of fluid each day than older children and adults. This makes them more dependent on adequate intake. Older children are also at risk for dehydration during exercise.
4. Health conditions that make infants and young children vulnerable to fluid deficits include increased respiratory rate during illness, fever, vomiting and diarrhea, and certain medical treatments.

 POWERPOINT SLIDES 20–27

Table 46–1. Electrolyte concentrations in body fluid compartments

 SUGGESTION FOR CLASSROOM ACTIVITIES

• Before class, assign students to do some Internet research on incidents of school-age athletes who have collapsed on a sports practice field. Use this as a framework for discussing why children are at risk for dehydration during exercise.

 SUGGESTION FOR CLINICAL ACTIVITIES

• Have students identify conditions in the child they are caring for, as well as medical treatments or procedures, that increase the child's risk for dehydration. Have students complete "Care Plan: Hyponatremic Dehydration in Breastfeeding" activity as review on *mynursingkit.com*

LEARNING OUTCOME 2

Identify regulatory mechanisms for fluid and electrolyte balance.

Concepts for Lecture

1. Conservation of fluid and electrolytes is primarily achieved through the kidney. Since infants and young children have immature kidneys, they are less able to conserve fluids and electrolytes.
2. Aldosterone causes the body to retain sodium and water. Antidiuretic hormone (ADH) causes the body to retain water.

 POWERPOINT SLIDES 28–32

 SUGGESTION FOR CLASSROOM ACTIVITIES

• When explaining the regulation of electrolytes and fluid balance, use examples that students can relate to. For example, ask them what their urine would look like if they had been febrile and vomiting for a day. Questions such as "How did your body know to concentrate your urine?" and "Would you expect the sodium level to be low, normal, or high in that urine?" can help them understand the physiology of the process.

 SUGGESTION FOR CLINICAL ACTIVITIES

• When caring for children with fluid and electrolyte imbalances, review laboratory tests that can help determine the degree of dehydration and the response to therapy.

LEARNING OUTCOME 3

Recognize threats to fluid and electrolyte balance in children.

Concepts for Lecture

1. Dehydration is one of the most common conditions during childhood, and there are three classifications of dehydration: isotonic, hypotonic, and hypertonic. Treatment is aimed at restoring fluid status. "Nursing Care Plan: The Child with Mild or Moderate Dehydration" and "Nursing Care Plan: The Child with Severe Dehydration" can be used to augment the discussion.
2. Extracellular fluid volume excess develops when there is too much fluid in the vascular and interstitial compartment. This may be caused by disease or by excessive IV fluid administration. Therapy focuses on treating the underlying cause and administration of diuretics.
3. Electrolytes are tightly regulated by the body, and are normally gained and lost in equal amounts in order to maintain a balance. Serum values reflect only the level of the electrolyte in the blood, and do not reflect the concentration of the electrolyte in other body compartments. Electrolyte abnormalities are reviewed in the corresponding slides.

LEARNING OUTCOME 4

Describe acid-base balance and recognize disruptions common in children.

Concepts for Lecture

1. The body tightly controls acid-base balance through several mechanisms, including the use of buffers, exhalation of carbon dioxide, and the excretion of metabolic acids.
2. Blood gases are used to evaluate the acid-base status.
3. The four major types of acid-base imbalance include respiratory acidosis, respiratory alkalosis, metabolic acidosis, and metabolic alkalosis.

PowerPoint Slides 33–60

SUGGESTION FOR CLASSROOM ACTIVITIES

- Before class, assign students to complete "Case Study: Dehydration and Fluid Calculation," available on *mynursingkit.com*. Use this assignment to frame your discussion of the treatment of dehydration.

SUGGESTION FOR CLINICAL ACTIVITIES

- Review the various devices used to gain access to the bloodstream, including peripheral IVs, central lines, and intraosseous lines. Discuss the care of the catheters and how sites and infusion rates vary in children.

PowerPoint Slides 61–79

Feature Box: Pathophysiology Illustrated: Buffer Responses to Acid and Base

Feature Box: Pathophysiology Illustrated: The Bicarbonate Buffer System

Feature Box: Pathophysiology Illustrated: The Kidneys and Metabolic Acids

ANIMATION

Acid-Base Balance

SUGGESTION FOR CLASSROOM ACTIVITIES

- During the discussion on acid-base balance, use the animation "Acid-Base Balance" on *mynursingkit.com* to enhance your teaching.

SUGGESTION FOR CLINICAL ACTIVITIES

- Students often have difficulty analyzing blood gases in the clinical setting. Take a group of students to the pediatric or neonatal intensive care units, where many blood gases are done. Examine the blood gases on a particular child to analyze trends and responses to treatments.

LEARNING OUTCOME 5

Analyze assessment findings to recognize fluid-electrolyte problems and acid-base imbalance in children.

Concepts for Lecture

1. A strategy for assessing children at risk for fluid and electrolyte imbalances is to perform a rapid risk assessment to see which factors are present. This strategy is reviewed in Tables 46–12 and 46–13.
2. Further assessment for fluid imbalances includes assessing weight changes, vascular volume interstitial volume, and cerebral function. Further assessment of electrolyte imbalance includes assessing serum electrolyte levels, skeletal muscle strength, neuromuscular excitability, gastrointestinal tract function, and cardiac rhythm. Tables 46-14 and 46-15 provide more details that may be useful references during the lecture.
3. Assessment findings with acid-base imbalances vary depending upon the particular imbalance.

 POWERPOINT SLIDES 80–90

Table 46–12. Risk factor assessment for fluid imbalances

Table 46–13. Risk factor assessment for electrolyte imbalances

Table 46–14. Summary of clinical assessment of fluid imbalances

Table 46–15. Summary of clinical assessment of electrolyte imbalances

 SUGGESTION FOR CLASSROOM ACTIVITIES

- To help students differentiate among various fluid, electrolyte, and acid-base assessment findings, create case studies of children with findings indicative of an imbalance. Challenge the class to identify the imbalance based upon the assessment findings you describe. You can also create a game out of this activity to make it competitive.

 SUGGESTION FOR CLINICAL ACTIVITIES

- Identify equipment in the clinical setting that is used in the monitoring and/or assessment of fluid, electrolyte, and acid-base imbalances (examples: scale, cardiac monitor, end-tidal carbon dioxide monitor, reflex hammer, etc.).

LEARNING OUTCOME 6

Describe appropriate nursing interventions for children experiencing fluid-electrolyte problems and acid-base imbalance.

Concepts for Lecture

1. Nursing interventions for children with fluid, electrolyte, and acid-base imbalances focus on correcting the underlying cause, monitoring for complications and response to therapy, and providing teaching to children and families.

 POWERPOINT SLIDES 91–108

 SUGGESTION FOR CLASSROOM ACTIVITIES

- For each electrolyte imbalance, have students draw a concept map that links the pathophysiology of the imbalance to the signs and symptoms, treatment, and nursing interventions. By understanding these linkages, students will better understand the monitoring and treatment of these imbalances.

 SUGGESTION FOR CLINICAL ACTIVITIES

- When caring for children with fluid and electrolyte imbalances, have students identify complications that could be life-threatening (e.g., shock, arrhythmias, seizures, etc.). Discuss the monitoring and treatment of these imbalances with the students.

GENERAL CHAPTER CONSIDERATIONS

1. Have students study and learn key terms listed at beginning of chapter.
2. Have students complete end-of-chapter exercises either in their book or on the MyNursingKit website.
3. Use the Classroom Response Questions provided in PowerPoint to assess students prior to lecture.

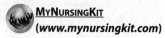

(www.mynursingkit.com)

- NCLEX RN® review questions
- Case Studies
- Care Plans
- Critical Concept Review
- Thinking Critically
- Weblinks
- Weblink applications
- Nursing Tools
- Audio Glossary
- Images and Tables Library

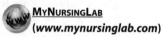

(www.mynursinglab.com)

- Knowledge Quick Check
- Pre/Posttests
- Customized study plans
- Images and Tables Library
- *Separate purchase*

CLINICAL SKILLS MANUAL

- *Separate purchase*

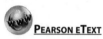

PEARSON eTEXT

- Students can search, highlight, take notes, and more all in electronic format
- *Separate purchase*

TESTBANK

Chapter 47
The Child with Alterations in Eye, Ear, Nose, and Throat Function

Learning Outcome 1

Identify anatomy, physiology, and pediatric differences in the eye, ear, nose, and throat of children and adolescents.

Concepts for Lecture

1. As newborns, infants have poor visual acuity. Their lens cannot accommodate, so they see best at a distance of about 8 inches. Their ability to distinguish details and colors is decreased. Visual acuity improves as the child grows, and by 6 to 7 years visual acuity is 20/20.
2. All newborns can hear, but the eustachian tube in infants is proportionately shorter, wider, and more horizontal than in adults. This anatomical configuration, as well as the fact that the tube briefly opens during sucking and yawning, predisposes infants to otitis media. As the child grows, the eustachian tube becomes more "adult like."
3. Infants are obligatory nose breathers until about 6 months of age. As a result, nasal discharge or edema can interfere with respiration and feeding. The tonsils are normally large in children, and decrease in size by around 10 years of age.

PowerPoint Slides 20–28

Table 47–1. Visually related developmental milestones

Video Clips

3D Ear/Ear Anatomy

Video Clips

3D Eye/Eye Anatomy

Suggestion for Classroom Activities

- Two of the videos on *mynursingkit.com*, "3D Ear/Ear Anatomy," and "3D Eye/Eye Anatomy," can provide visual references as you discuss these concepts.

Suggestion for Clinical Activities

- Students often have difficulty learning to examine the eyes and ears of children, since children are often uncooperative with the exam. When students are working in areas where children are sedated (such as the intensive care unit), there are often good opportunities to help students develop these assessment skills.

Learning Outcome 2

Describe abnormalities of the eyes, ears, nose, throat, and mouth in children.

Concepts for Lecture

1. Common eye abnormalities in children include conjunctivitis, cellulitis, visual disorders, and injuries to the eye.
2. Common ear abnormalities in children include otitis media, otitis externa, and hearing impairment.
3. Common disorders of the nose, throat, and mouth include epistaxis, nasopharyngitis, sinusitis, tonsillitis, adenoiditis, and trauma to the mouth and teeth.

PowerPoint Slides 29–65

Figure 47–1. Acute conjunctivitis

Figure 47–4. Acute otitis media

Figure 47–5. Otitis media with effusion

Figure 47–6. Signs of otitis media

Animation

Middle Ear Dynamics

SUGGESTIONS FOR CLASSROOM ACTIVITIES

- Watch the animation "Middle Ear Dynamics" and the video "Otitis Media" to augment your discussion of this outcome.
- Have students complete the activity on *mynursingkit.com,* "Case Study: Otitis Media."

SUGGESTION FOR CLINICAL ACTIVITIES

- Many of the preceding disorders are most commonly diagnosed in the outpatient setting. Consider assigning students to an outpatient acute care clinic or a pediatrician's office in order to give them the opportunity to observe and care for children with these disorders.

LEARNING OUTCOME 3

Plan for screening programs and identification of children with vision and hearing abnormalities.

Concepts for Lecture

1. Early identification of vision and hearing deficits through screening is critical in order to prevent further vision and hearing loss.

POWERPOINT SLIDES 66–69

SUGGESTION FOR CLINICAL ACTIVITIES

- Assign students to work with a school nurse at a local elementary school and have the students assist with vision and hearing screenings. Recommend that students review Skills 9–18 through 9–19, "Visual Acuity Screening" available in the *Clinical Skills Manual* before attending the screenings.

LEARNING OUTCOME 4

Plan nursing care for children with vision or hearing impairments.

Concepts for Lecture

1. Nursing interventions for children with vision impairment include encouraging the use of all senses, promoting socialization, and encouraging normality.
2. Nursing interventions for children with hearing impairment include techniques for communicating with deaf children, awareness of hearing aids used by children, and facilitating interpreters.

POWERPOINT SLIDES 70–75

SUGGESTION FOR CLASSROOM ACTIVITIES

- Before class, assign students to review the websites regarding cochlear implants listed in the Weblinks available on *mynursingkit.com.* Use this activity as a basis for discussing nursing interventions for children with hearing impairments.

SUGGESTION FOR CLINICAL ACTIVITIES

- Ask a sign language interpreter or audiologist to attend a clinical conference in order to discuss practical interventions for children with hearing impairments.

LEARNING OUTCOME 5

Use latest recommendations when implementing care and teaching for children with abnormalities of eyes, ears, nose, throat, and mouth.

Concepts for Lecture

1. Because so many children are affected by disorders of the eyes, ears, nose, throat, and mouth, recommendations regarding identification and treatment are routinely updated. Nurses are in a unique position to implement and educate families about these recommendations.

LEARNING OUTCOME 6

Integrate preventive and treatment principles when implementing care for children related to eyes, ears, nose, and throat.

Concepts for Lecture

1. Many injuries to the eyes, ears, nose, throat, and mouth are preventable. Common prevention strategies are reviewed.

 VIDEO CLIPS

Nursing in Action: Ophthalmic, Otic, and Nasal Medication Administration

 VIDEO CLIPS

Nursing in Action: Child with a Sore Throat

 POWERPOINT SLIDES 76–80

 SUGGESTIONS FOR CLASSROOM ACTIVITIES

- During class, have students read "Evidence-Based Nursing: Nursing Role in Vision Screening and Follow-up." Use the Critical Thinking questions to have a discussion about how nurses could apply this information to practice.
- Show the two "Nursing in Action" videos available on *mynursingkit.com*

 SUGGESTION FOR CLINICAL ACTIVITIES

- While in the clinical setting, encourage students to talk with physicians about their views regarding the use of antibiotics to treat otitis media.

 POWERPOINT SLIDES 81–84

 SUGGESTION FOR CLASSROOM ACTIVITIES

- Remind students that any organic object that is stuck in the ear or nose will expand due to the moisture present in the cavity. You can demonstrate this in class by taking a pea, peanut, or other common object and placing it in a glass of water. Students will note that it swells and expands over time.

 SUGGESTION FOR CLINICAL ACTIVITIES

- Assign students to observe in the pediatric emergency room, where many injuries to the eyes, ears, nose, and throat are seen.

General Chapter Considerations

1. Have students study and learn key terms listed at beginning of chapter.
2. Have students complete end-of-chapter exercises either in their book or on the MyNursingKit website.
3. Use the Classroom Response Questions provided in PowerPoint to assess students prior to lecture.

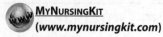

MyNursingKit
(*www.mynursingkit.com*)

- NCLEX RN® review questions
- Case Studies
- Care Plans
- Critical Concept Review
- Thinking Critically
- Weblinks
- Weblink applications
- Nursing Tools
- Audio Glossary
- Images and Tables Library

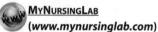

MyNursingLab
(*www.mynursinglab.com*)

- Knowledge Quick Check
- Pre/Posttests
- Customized study plans
- Images and Tables Library
- *Separate purchase*

Clinical Skills Manual

- *Separate purchase*

Pearson eText

- Students can search, highlight, take notes, and more all in electronic format
- *Separate purchase*

Testbank

CHAPTER 48
THE CHILD WITH ALTERATIONS IN RESPIRATORY FUNCTION

LEARNING OUTCOME 1

Describe unique characteristics of the pediatric respiratory system anatomy and physiology and apply that information to the care of children with respiratory conditions.

Concepts for Lecture

1. A child's respiratory tract continues to grow and change until about 12 years of age. There are significant differences between the adult and pediatric airway.
2. The child's upper airway is short and narrow, which increases the potential for obstruction. A child's little finger is a good estimate for the diameter of his or her airway size. There is an inverse relationship between airway diameter and resistance: The narrower the airway is, the greater the airway resistance.
3. The child's lower airway also develops throughout childhood. The alveoli change size and shape and increase in number until puberty. This increases the area available for gas exchange. Smooth muscles of the bronchi and bronchioles develop during the first year of life. Until children are about 6 years of age, the intercostal muscles are immature and the diaphragm is the primary muscle used for ventilation. The cartilaginous ribs are very flexible, which causes retractions that worsen during respiratory distress.

 POWERPOINT SLIDES 20–30

Feature Box: As Children Grow: Airway Development

Feature Box: As Children Grow: Trachea Position

Feature Box: Pathophysiology Illustrated: Retraction Sites

 ANIMATION

CO_2 and O_2 Transport

 ANIMATION

Gas Exchange

 SUGGESTION FOR CLASSROOM ACTIVITIES

- Show the animations "CO_2 and O_2 Transport" and "Gas Exchange" available on *mynursingkit.com*. How are infants able to sustain life-sustaining gas exchange if they have fewer alveoli than adults?

 SUGGESTION FOR CLINICAL ACTIVITIES

- Endotracheal tubes (ETTs) closely estimate the size of a child's airway. Visit the emergency department, pediatric intensive care unit, or pediatric operating room to view the various sizes of ETTs available. This gives students a visual reference to the size of a child's airway.

LEARNING OUTCOME 2

Identify the assessment guidelines for a child with a respiratory condition.

Concepts for Lecture

1. Since children with respiratory distress can quickly progress to respiratory failure, it is important to assess these children accurately. Details about these assessment guidelines are listed in Table 48-1, "Assessment Guidelines for a Child in Respiratory Distress."

 POWERPOINT SLIDES 31–32

Table 48–1. Assessment guidelines for a child in respiratory distress

 SUGGESTION FOR CLASSROOM ACTIVITIES

- List signs and symptoms of varying degrees of respiratory distress on the board and have students pick out which symptoms are mild and which ones are severe (example: sitting in tripod position versus sitting straight up).

LEARNING OUTCOME 3

List the different respiratory conditions and injuries that can cause respiratory distress in infants and children.

Concepts for Lecture

1. Conditions that can cause respiratory distress in children can be divided into two categories: acute and chronic.
2. Injuries of the respiratory system include smoke inhalation, blunt chest trauma, pulmonary contusion, and pneumothorax.
3. All of the above conditions may lead to respiratory failure, which occurs when the body can no longer maintain effective gas exchange.

LEARNING OUTCOME 4

Assess the child's respiratory signs and symptoms to distinguish between respiratory distress and respiratory failure and describe the appropriate nursing care.

Concepts for Lecture

1. Respiratory distress can lead to respiratory failure if it is not recognized and treated promptly. Refer to Table 48-1 and "Clinical Manifestations: Respiratory Failure and Imminent Respiratory Arrest" during this part of the lecture.
2. Mild respiratory distress has signs that indicate the child is attempting to compensate.
3. Moderate respiratory distress marks the beginning of initial decompensation.
4. Severe respiratory distress signals that respiratory arrest is imminent.

POWERPOINT SLIDES 33–41

Feature Box: Pathophysiology Illustrated: Pneumothorax

VIDEO CLIPS

SIDS

SUGGESTION FOR CLASSROOM ACTIVITIES

• There are numerous disorders discussed in this chapter. Have students group together in pairs and assign each pairing a brief overview of a disorder to present to the whole class.

SUGGESTION FOR CLINICAL ACTIVITIES

• Have students role-play what to do in the event of a respiratory arrest. Correct use of a mask and Ambu-bag can be reviewed.

POWERPOINT SLIDES 42–46

Table 48–1. Assessment guidelines for a child in respiratory distress

VIDEO CLIPS

Pediatric Respiratory Emergency Management

SUGGESTION FOR CLASSROOM ACTIVITIES

• Demonstrate each of the three degrees of respiratory distress described and have students identify which phase of distress you are in. Then have them identify nursing interventions that are appropriate for each level.

SUGGESTION FOR CLINICAL ACTIVITIES

• Discuss medications commonly used to treat respiratory diseases in children. Administration and monitoring may be discussed.

LEARNING OUTCOME 5

Distinguish between conditions of the upper respiratory tract that cause respiratory distress.

Concepts for Lecture

1. Common causes of respiratory distress involving the upper respiratory tract include foreign-body aspiration, croup, laryngotracheobronchitis, epiglottitis, and bacterial tracheitis.

 POWERPOINT SLIDES 47–58

Figure 48–1. Aspirated foreign body

Figure 48–2. Epiglottitis

 SUGGESTION FOR CLASSROOM ACTIVITIES

- Bring various items to class that are often associated with foreign-body aspiration and pass them around during the discussion on FBA. Remind students how to estimate the size of a child's airway.

 SUGGESTION FOR CLINICAL ACTIVITIES

- Many clients with respiratory disorders are monitored with pulse oximeters. Discuss the limitations of pulse oximetry as a monitoring device. Students may review "Skill 14–2: Oxygen Saturation: Pulse Oximetry" in the *Clinical Skills Manual*.

LEARNING OUTCOME 6

Distinguish between conditions of the lower respiratory tract that cause illness in children.

Concepts for Lecture

1. Common causes of conditions affecting the lower respiratory tract include bronchitis, bronchiolitis, pneumonia, and tuberculosis.

 POWERPOINT SLIDES 59–63

 SUGGESTION FOR CLASSROOM ACTIVITIES

- Provide copies of line drawings of the basic pediatric airway. Divide students into groups and have them sketch in a drawing representing the pathophysiology of a respiratory disease. Have groups share their results with the class.

SUGGESTION FOR CLINICAL ACTIVITIES

- Ask students to compare the differences in respiratory diseases between children and adults. For example, how is pneumonia in an infant different from pneumonia in an adult? What needs to be monitored? How is it treated?

LEARNING OUTCOME 7

Develop a hospital-based nursing care plan for a child with a common acute respiratory condition.

Concepts for Lecture

1. For this outcome, bronchopulmonary dysplasia (BPD) will serve as the model nursing care plan for acute respiratory conditions. Students may also refer to "Nursing Care Plan: The Child with Bronchiolitis" in the textbook.
2. Common nursing interventions for any child hospitalized with an acute respiratory condition include monitoring, supporting the family, and teaching about the disease process.

 POWERPOINT SLIDES 64–72

 SUGGESTION FOR CLASSROOM ACTIVITIES

- Ask students to think about why infants and young children with bronchiolitis tend to require more aggressive treatment than older children and adults with bronchiolitis. What makes the disease process different in these two groups? Assign "Care Plan: The Child with Cystic Fibrosis" from *mynursingkit.com* for review after class.

LEARNING OUTCOME 8

Develop a school-based nursing care plan for the child with asthma.

Concepts for Lecture

1. Since asthma is a very common chronic disease during childhood, many children in the school setting have a diagnosis of asthma. Nursing management in the school focuses on monitoring for exacerbations and teaching the child about the disease process.

LEARNING OUTCOME 9

Develop a home nursing care plan for the child with a cystic fibrosis.

Concepts for Lecture

1. Cystic fibrosis requires a significant amount of time, energy, and knowledge to manage in the home. Families need education and coordination of care from nurses.

 SUGGESTION FOR CLINICAL ACTIVITIES

- When a student is caring for an infant with bronchiolitis, discuss the relationship between suctioning the nose and feeding times. A patent nasal passage greatly increases the infant's ability to feed.

 POWERPOINT SLIDES 73–75

 SUGGESTION FOR CLASSROOM ACTIVITIES

- Before class, have students design an educational brochure (or handout or poster) for school-age children explaining the correct use of peak flow meters and inhalers. Have the students share their teaching projects with the class.

 SUGGESTION FOR CLINICAL ACTIVITIES

- When students are assigned to be with a school nurse, have them review the school nurse's care plan for a child with asthma.

 POWERPOINT SLIDES 76–79

 SUGGESTION FOR CLASSROOM ACTIVITIES

- Have students make a list of all the daily required medications and respiratory treatments required for a child with CF. How much time would a family need to allow to complete all the treatments each day?

 SUGGESTION FOR CLINICAL ACTIVITIES

- Students often find the psychosocial component of chronic illness difficult to approach with a child and family. When a student has a client with CF, role-play methods the student can use to address the psychosocial issues surrounding this chronic illness with the child and family.

GENERAL CHAPTER CONSIDERATIONS

1. Have students study and learn key terms listed at beginning of chapter.
2. Have students complete end-of-chapter exercises either in their book or on the MyNursingKit website.
3. Use the Classroom Response Questions provided in PowerPoint to assess students prior to lecture.

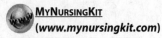

MyNursingKit (*www.mynursingkit.com*)

- NCLEX RN® review questions
- Case Studies
- Care Plans
- Critical Concept Review
- Thinking Critically
- Weblinks
- Weblink applications
- Nursing Tools
- Audio Glossary
- Images and Tables Library

MyNursingLab (*www.mynursinglab.com*)

- Knowledge Quick Check
- Pre/Posttests
- Customized study plans
- Images and Tables Library
- *Separate purchase*

CLINICAL SKILLS MANUAL

- *Separate purchase*

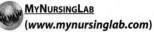

PEARSON eTEXT

- Students can search, highlight, take notes, and more all in electronic format
- *Separate purchase*

TESTBANK

CHAPTER 49
THE CHILD WITH ALTERATIONS IN CARDIOVASCULAR FUNCTION

LEARNING OUTCOME 1

Describe the anatomy and physiology of the cardiovascular system focusing on the flow of blood and action of the heart valves.

Concepts for Lecture

1. Significant cardiovascular changes occur as newborns transition from intrauterine to extrauterine life.
2. In order to understand the anatomy and pathophysiology of congenital heart defects, it is very important to understand the normal anatomy of the heart.
3. Normal vital signs change during childhood. For example, normal blood pressure starts low during infancy and rises as the child grows.
4. Infants have very little reserve in terms of oxygenation and cardiac output. Infants and children respond to severe hypoxemia with bradycardia—thus, bradycardia is a significant warning sign of impending cardiac arrest.

 POWERPOINT SLIDES 19–25

 ANIMATION

Blood Pressure

 SUGGESTION FOR CLASSROOM ACTIVITIES

- Have students pretend that they are a single red blood cell, and have them make a list of how they travel through the body. This helps students to visualize the cardiovascular system in a different way than just by looking at a picture.

 SUGGESTION FOR CLINICAL ACTIVITIES

- Discuss how interventions for bradycardia differ in children compared to adults, and how hypoxia relates to bradycardia.

LEARNING OUTCOME 2

Describe the pathophysiology associated with congenital heart defects with increased pulmonary circulation, decreased pulmonary circulation, mixed defects, and obstructed systemic blood flow.

Concepts for Lecture

1. Congenital heart defects that increase pulmonary blood flow include patent ductus arteriosus, atrial septal defect, ventricular septal defect, and atrioventricular canal defect. Refer to Table 49-3 for details.
2. Congenital heart defects that decrease pulmonary blood flow include pulmonic stenosis, tetralogy of Fallot, and pulmonary or tricuspid atresia. Refer to Table 49-5 for details.
3. Mixed congenital heart defects include transposition of the great arteries (TGA), truncus arteriosus, and total anomalous pulmonary venous return (TAPVR). Infant survival is dependent upon the mixing of systemic and pulmonary blood. Refer to Table 49-6 for details.
4. Obstructive congenital heart defects include aortic stenosis (AS), coarctation of the aorta (COA), and hypoplastic left heart syndrome (HLHS). Refer to Table 49-7 for details.

 POWERPOINT SLIDES 26–62

Table 49–3. Pathophysiology, clinical manifestations, and clinical therapy for heart defects that increase pulmonary blood flow (and figures therein)

Table 49–5. Pathophysiology, clinical manifestations, and clinical therapy for defects with decreased pulmonary blood flow (and figures therein)

Table 49–6. Pathophysiology, clinical manifestations, and clinical therapy for mixed defects (and figures therein)

Table 49–7. Pathophysiology, clinical manifestations, and clinical therapy for defects that obstruct the systemic blood flow (and figures therein)

LEARNING OUTCOME 3

Develop a nursing care plan for the infant with a congenital heart defect cared for at home prior to corrective surgery.

Concepts for Lecture

1. The nursing care plan can be applied to families caring at home for children who are awaiting corrective surgery. Refer to "Nursing Care Plan: The Child with Congestive Heart Failure Being Cared for at Home" for details.

LEARNING OUTCOME 4

Develop a nursing care plan for the child undergoing open-heart surgery.

Concepts for Lecture

1. Assessment of the infant or child who has undergone surgical repair includes a head-to-toe physical assessment, as well as assessing the psychosocial and developmental aspects. Refer to Table 49–4 for details regarding assessment.
2. Nursing diagnoses may relate to pain, breathing, fluid volume, and infection.
3. Planning and implementation include pain management, promoting respiratory function, managing fluids and nutrition, encouraging activity, and planning for discharge. Home teaching is also important.
4. Evaluation is completed to assess the effectiveness of interventions.

SUGGESTION FOR CLASSROOM ACTIVITIES

- Many students learn by seeing and doing, so have the students create these heart defects. After dividing them into groups, distribute blank paper, colored markers, and Play-Dough. Assign each group to either draw or sculpt (using Play-Dough) a heart defect and then present it to the class. Hint: Use red for oxygenated blood, blue for deoxygenated blood, and purple for mixed blood. Red and blue Play-Dough can be mixed together to create purple.

SUGGESTION FOR CLINICAL ACTIVITIES

- Identify teaching resources available in the clinical setting for use in teaching children and families about different congenital heart defects.

POWERPOINT SLIDES 63–70

SUGGESTION FOR CLASSROOM ACTIVITIES

- Challenge students to think about the relationship between growth and congenital heart defects. Why is growth so challenging for infants with heart defects? Why is it so important for growth to occur? How does growth relate to the timing and potential success of their surgery?

SUGGESTION FOR CLINICAL ACTIVITIES

- Have students develop a teaching plan for the family who will care for a child at home who is awaiting corrective surgery. Include "Skill 15–2: Inserting and Removing a Nasogastric Tube" and "Skill 15–3: Administering a Gavage Feeding" in the *Clinical Skills Manual* if the family will be performing these procedures at home.

POWERPOINT SLIDES 71–76

Table 49–4. Guidelines for assessment of the child with a cardiac condition

SUGGESTION FOR CLASSROOM ACTIVITIES

- Before class, assign students to review "Case Study: Newborn after Heart Surgery," available on *mynursingkit.com*. Use this case study as the basis for discussion during the development of this care plan. Assign "Care Plan: Pediatric Heart Transplant" from *mynursingkit.com* for homework.

SUGGESTION FOR CLINICAL ACTIVITIES

- Assign students to the pediatric intensive care unit to directly observe the nursing care of an infant or child after open-heart surgery.

LEARNING OUTCOME 5

Recognize the signs and symptoms of congestive heart failure in an infant and child.

Concepts for Lecture

1. Congestive heart failure (CHF) occurs when cardiac output cannot keep up with the body's circulatory and metabolic demands. CHF may result from congenital heart defects, problems with heart contractility, and disease processes that require high cardiac output. CHF may also result from acquired heart diseases such as cardiomyopathy or Kawasaki disease.
2. Early signs of CHF in infants include tiring during feeding, weight loss, diaphoresis, and frequent infections. Early signs of CHF in children include exercise intolerance, dyspnea, abdominal pain, and peripheral edema. Late signs of CHF include tachypnea and other respiratory symptoms, tachycardia, and cardiomegaly. "Clinical Manifestations: Congestive Heart Failure" is a good reference for this topic.

LEARNING OUTCOME 6

Develop a nursing care plan for a child with congestive heart failure.

Concepts for Lecture

1. Assessment of the infant or child with CHF includes a head-to-toe physical assessment, as well as assessing the family and developmental aspects.
2. Nursing diagnoses may include decreased cardiac output, increased fluid volume, risk for impaired skin integrity, imbalanced nutrition, and compromised family coping. Refer to "Nursing Care Plan: The Child Hospitalized with Congestive Heart Failure" for details.
3. Planning and implementation include administration of medications, maintaining oxygenation, promoting rest, fostering development, providing adequate nutrition, and providing support and discharge teaching.
4. Evaluation is completed to assess the effectiveness of interventions.

LEARNING OUTCOME 7

Differentiate between the acquired heart diseases that occur during childhood.

Concepts for Lecture

1. Rheumatic fever is an inflammatory disorder of the connective tissue that follows an initial infection by some strains of group A beta-hemolytic streptococci. The heart, joints, brain, and skin tissues are affected.

POWERPOINT SLIDES 77–83

ANIMATION

Congenital Heart Defects

SUGGESTION FOR CLASSROOM ACTIVITIES

- Show the animation "Congenital Heart Defects," available on *mynursingkit.com*. This helps illustrate the relationship between CHF and congenital heart defects.

SUGGESTION FOR CLINICAL ACTIVITIES

- When caring for a child at risk of CHF, discuss specific signs and symptoms that should be assessed and monitored based on the child's age. Compare these signs and symptoms to those of adults with CHF.

POWERPOINT SLIDES 84–90

Feature Box: Drug Guide: Drugs Used to Treat Congestive Heart Failure

ANIMATION

Digoxin

SUGGESTION FOR CLASSROOM ACTIVITIES

- When discussing medications used to treat CHF, show the animation "Digoxin," located on *mynursingkit.com*. This helps students visualize the action of the drug.

SUGGESTION FOR CLINICAL ACTIVITIES

- Have students discuss how to administer digoxin, including monitoring of blood levels and other associated labs, dosing, assessment of the child, and signs of toxicity

POWERPOINT SLIDES 91–103

Figure 49–7. This child shows many of the signs of the acute stage of Kawasaki disease

2. Infective endocarditis is an inflammation of the lining, valves, and arterial vessels of the heart. It may be caused by bacterial, enterococci, and fungal infections. Valvular damage from the infection may result in congestive heart failure.

3. Kawasaki disease is an acute systemic vascular inflammatory illness that is the leading cause of acquired heart disease in children. The etiology is unknown, although it is believed that there is an infectious trigger in genetically predisposed children. The disease affects the small- and medium-sized arteries, including the coronary arteries.

LEARNING OUTCOME 8

List strategies to reduce the child's risk of adult onset cardiovascular disease.

Concepts for Lecture

1. Health promotion activities that impact cardiovascular disease during adulthood begin during childhood. The nurse can work with families and children to discuss strategies for developing healthy eating habits, encouraging physical activity, and not smoking.

LEARNING OUTCOME 9

Describe the development of hypovolemic shock and nursing management of the condition.

Concepts for Lecture

1. Hypovolemic shock occurs when there is inadequate tissue and organ perfusion resulting from a loss of fluid in the intravascular compartment. It is typically caused by a severely depleted blood volume or dehydration.

Audio: Heart Sounds Audio Series:

- Heart Sound: Normal Heart Sound: Infant—4 months
- Heart Sound: Normal Heart Sound: Child—12 years old
- Heart Sound: Normal Heart Sound: Child—100 Beats per Minute
- Heart Sound: Physiological S2 split: Child—12 years old
- Heart Sound: Continuous Murmur caused by Patent Ductus Arteriosus
- Heart Sound: Non-continuous Systolic Murmur/Hypertrophic Cardiomyopathy
- Heart Sound: Normal Physiological Arrhythmia

SUGGESTION FOR CLASSROOM ACTIVITIES

- Use the audio series "Heart Sounds" on *mynursingkit.com* to discuss how heart murmurs may appear or change in the presence of infective endocarditis.

SUGGESTION FOR CLINICAL ACTIVITIES

- Aspirin always comes in tablet, or solid, form. Have students demonstrate how they would administer aspirin to a toddler with Kawasaki disease.

POWERPOINT SLIDES 104–108

SUGGESTION FOR CLASSROOM ACTIVITIES

- Currently, only certain with certain risk factors are screened for dyslipidemia. Discuss the concept of screening tests, and ask the class why every child is not given a blood test. Economics of screening and prevalence of disease can be discussed.

SUGGESTION FOR CLINICAL ACTIVITIES

- Have students identify or develop teaching materials that can be used to teach families and children the health promotion concepts that help prevent heart disease during adulthood.

POWERPOINT SLIDES 109–114

Feature Box: Pathophysiology Illustrated: Hypovolemic Shock

Feature Box: Clinical Manifestations: Hypovolemic Shock

- Divide students into groups and provide each group with a blank overhead transparency and colored markers. Have them draw a concept map showing the pathophysiology of hypovolemic shock. Share the concept maps with the entire class.

SUGGESTION FOR CLINICAL ACTIVITIES

- While caring for a child with shock, discuss how laboratory values can reflect end-organ perfusion. Examples include liver function tests, BUN and creatinine, and lactate levels.

MyNursingKit
(*www.mynursingkit.com*)

- NCLEX RN® review questions
- Case Studies
- Care Plans
- Critical Concept Review
- Thinking Critically
- Weblinks
- Weblink applications
- Nursing Tools
- Audio Glossary
- Images and Tables Library

MyNursingLab
(*www.mynursinglab.com*)

- Knowledge Quick Check
- Pre/Posttests
- Customized study plans
- Images and Tables Library
- *Separate purchase*

CLINICAL SKILLS MANUAL

- *Separate purchase*

PEARSON eTEXT

- Students can search, highlight, take notes, and more all in electronic format
- *Separate purchase*

TESTBANK

GENERAL CHAPTER CONSIDERATIONS

1. Have students study and learn key terms listed at beginning of chapter.
2. Have students complete end-of-chapter exercises either in their book or on the MyNursingKit website.
3. Use the Classroom Response Questions provided in PowerPoint to assess students prior to lecture.

CHAPTER 50
THE CHILD WITH ALTERATIONS IN IMMUNE FUNCTION

LEARNING OUTCOME 1

Describe the structure and function of the immune system and apply that knowledge to the care of children with immunologic disorders.

Concepts for Lecture

1. The primary function of the immune system is to recognize foreign substances in the body and to eliminate these foreign substances as efficiently as possible.
2. Antibodies are found in serum, body fluids, and certain tissues. Antibodies are a type of protein called immunoglobulins, of which there are five types.
3. The primary immune response occurs once an antigen invades the body and antibodies are reactive to specific antigens. This is the primary response and occurs within 3 days. Once the antigen has been encountered, secondary immune response occurs (usually within 24 hours) after each subsequent encounter.

 POWERPOINT SLIDES 19–25

Table 50–1. Classes of immunoglobulins

Feature Box: Pathophysiology Illustrated: Primary Immune Response

 SUGGESTION FOR CLASSROOM ACTIVITIES

- When discussing immune response, use the analogy of a war, including soldiers (antibodies), the enemy (antigens), supply lines (vasodilation), and so on.

 SUGGESTION FOR CLINICAL ACTIVITIES

- Discuss why newborns and young children are more at risk for infection than older children and adults.

LEARNING OUTCOME 2

Identify infection control measures to prevent the spread of infection in children with an immunodeficiency.

Concepts for Lecture

1. There are numerous nursing interventions that can be used to prevent infection in children with an immunodeficiency, including handwashing, standard and transmission-based precautions, sterile technique, and avoiding contact with infected individuals.

 POWERPOINT SLIDES 26–28

 SUGGESTION FOR CLASSROOM ACTIVITIES

- Have students list which vaccines are live virus vaccines and which ones are not.

 SUGGESTION FOR CLINICAL ACTIVITIES

- Review the equipment available in the local clinical setting that can be used to prevent transmission of infection.

LEARNING OUTCOME 3

Develop a nursing care plan in partnership with the family for a child with human immunodeficiency virus (HIV infection).

Concepts for Lecture

1. Prevention of the spread of HIV is important, especially for neonates whose mothers have HIV. Proper disposal of used needles and using standard precautions can also help prevent spreading HIV.
2. Prevention of further infection is important for children with HIV. Interventions include frequent handwashing, limiting exposure to infected people, and following a modified immunization schedule.

 POWERPOINT SLIDES 29–37

 ANIMATION

HIV Infection/Transmission

 VIDEO CLIPS

AIDS/HIV

3. Promote adherence to the medication regimen, as nonadherence may result in increased morbidity and mortality.
4. Children with HIV infection are at risk for pneumonia, so promotion of respiratory function is important in preventing infections.
5. Children with HIV infection are at risk for failure to thrive. Adequate nutritional intake can be promoted by encouraging parents to provide nutritious meals and supplementing vitamins.
6. Emotional support should be provided to both the family and the child. Although the survival and long-term outlook for children with HIV has greatly improved, there is still a social stigma involved with the disease.

LEARNING OUTCOME 4

Describe nursing management for the child with systemic lupus erythematosus or juvenile arthritis.

Concepts for Lecture

1. Systemic lupus erythematosus (SLE) and juvenile arthritis (JA) (classically known as juvenile rheumatoid arthritis) are both chronic autoimmune disorders. SLE involves the deposition of antigen-antibody complexes into connective tissue, triggering an inflammatory response. Small blood vessels, glomeruli, joints, spleen, and heart valves are commonly affected. JA involves the joints and is characterized by decreased mobility, swelling, and pain.
2. Nursing interventions that are common to both diseases include promoting adequate nutrition, managing flare-ups, managing side effects of medication, promoting rest and comfort, and providing emotional support.
3. Nursing interventions specific to SLE include promoting skin integrity, preventing infection, and maintaining fluid balance.
4. Nursing interventions specific to JA include promoting improved mobility.

LEARNING OUTCOME 5

Describe exposure prevention measures for the child with latex allergy.

Concepts for Lecture

1. Latex allergy is increasingly common, as sources of latex products have risen in the past few years. Healthcare workers and clients are at risk. Table 50–6 is a good reference. Symptoms of latex allergy range from mild topical reactions to full anaphylaxis.
2. Exposure to latex must be prevented in a child with known latex allergies. This involves removing all sources of latex from the child's environment, as well as teaching parents what to do in case of a reaction.

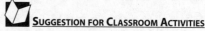 **SUGGESTION FOR CLASSROOM ACTIVITIES**

- During the discussion on HIV, show the animation "HIV Infection/Transmission" and the video "AIDS/HIV," available on *mynursingkit.com*

 SUGGESTION FOR CLINICAL ACTIVITIES

- Assign students to the infectious disease clinic to observe the outpatient management of children with HIV and AIDS.

 POWERPOINT SLIDES 38–44

 ANIMATION

Methotrexate

 SUGGESTION FOR CLASSROOM ACTIVITIES

- Methotrexate may be used to treat both SLE and JA. Show the animation "Methotrexate," available on *mynursingkit.com* and discuss how the drug modulates these disease processes.

 SUGGESTION FOR CLINICAL ACTIVITIES

- Attend a local support group, clinic, or active Web chat for children with chronic inflammatory disease such as SLE or JA.

 POWERPOINT SLIDES 45–51

Table 50–6. Sources of latex in the home and community with recommended alternatives

 SUGGESTION FOR CLASSROOM ACTIVITIES

- Using Table 50–6, have students make a list of latex-containing products that are in their own houses. This will help to increase their awareness of various products that contain latex.

 SUGGESTION FOR CLINICAL ACTIVITIES

- Have students search the clinical unit for products that contain latex. Many hospitals have adopted a latex-free environment. If so, have students identify various sources of latex that families may bring to the hospital (e.g., latex balloons, home feeding nipples, home pacifiers, etc.).

LEARNING OUTCOME 6

Apply nursing interventions and prevention measures for the child experiencing other hypersensitivity reactions.

Concepts for Lecture

1. Many children have allergies, and allergic reactions can range from mild to severe. Allergens are substances that trigger a reaction and can be inhaled, ingested, or absorbed.
2. There are several nursing interventions that should be implemented for the child with hypersensitivity reactions, including careful assessment, teaching how to minimize or prevent exposure, and allergy-proofing the home

GENERAL CHAPTER CONSIDERATIONS

1. Have students study and learn key terms listed at beginning of chapter.
2. Have students complete end-of-chapter exercises either in their book or on the MyNursingKit website.
3. Use the Classroom Response Questions provided in PowerPoint to assess students prior to lecture.

  POWERPOINT SLIDES 52–59

Table 50–5. Characteristic findings in children with allergies

 SUGGESTION FOR CLASSROOM ACTIVITIES

- Before class, assign students to gather information about how to "allergy-proof" a home. Use their findings to augment the discussion of the topic during the lecture.

 SUGGESTION FOR CLINICAL ACTIVITIES

- Assign students to spend a day in an allergy clinic or office. The students may observe different types of testing and education for specific allergies. The student could provide a detailed case report of a child observed that day.

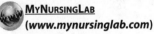 **MYNURSINGKIT** (*www.mynursingkit.com*)

- NCLEX RN® review questions
- Case Studies
- Care Plans
- Critical Concept Review
- Thinking Critically
- Weblinks
- Weblink applications
- Nursing Tools
- Audio Glossary
- Images and Tables Library

 MYNURSINGLAB (*www.mynursinglab.com*)

- Knowledge Quick Check
- Pre/Posttests
- Customized study plans
- Images and Tables Library
- *Separate purchase*

CLINICAL SKILLS MANUAL

- *Separate purchase*

 PEARSON ETEXT

- Students can search, highlight, take notes, and more all in electronic format
- *Separate purchase*

TESTBANK

CHAPTER 51
THE CHILD WITH ALTERATIONS IN HEMATOLOGIC FUNCTION

LEARNING OUTCOME 1

Describe the function of red blood cells, white blood cells, and platelets.

Concepts for Lecture

1. Red blood cells transport oxygen from the lungs to the tissues, and return carbon dioxide back to the lungs.
2. White blood cells are composed of five different types of cells, with functions primarily involved in immunity, phagocytosis, and inflammation. White blood cells essentially aid in protecting the body.
3. Platelets function as part of the clotting cascade to stop bleeding.

 POWERPOINT SLIDES 21–29

Figure 51–1. Types of blood cells

Table 51–2. White blood cells and their functions

Activity: Circulatory System

Activity: Types of Blood Cells

 SUGGESTION FOR CLASSROOM ACTIVITIES

- Have students view and try to complete the activities "Circulatory System" and "Types of Blood Cells," available on *mynursingkit.com* before discussing the functions of red blood cells, white blood cells, and platelets. Have them repeat the activity after the discussion to reinforce what they learned in class.

SUGGESTION FOR CLINICAL ACTIVITIES

- Many hospitalized children have a complete blood count (CBC) performed during their illness. Have students analyze the lab results and discuss abnormal values and significant normal values. Students can also discuss the various ranges of normal lab values based on the age of the child (for example, a normal WBC of a newborn versus an adolescent).

LEARNING OUTCOME 2

Discuss the pathophysiology and clinical manifestations of the major disorders of red blood cells affecting the pediatric population.

Concepts for Lecture

1. Iron-deficiency anemia is the most common type of anemia and the most common nutritional deficiency in children. Infants and children who are malnourished or who do not have adequate iron intake are at risk, as well as children who have chronic blood loss. Clinical manifestations include pallor, fatigue, and irritability.
2. Normocytic anemia occurs as a result of numerous inflammatory and infectious conditions. Clinical manifestations are similar to iron-deficiency anemia, although hepatomegaly and splenomegaly may also be present.

 POWERPOINT SLIDES 30–49

Feature Box: Pathophysiology Illustrated: Sickle Cell Anemia

ANIMATION

Sickle Cell Anemia

3. Sickle-cell anemia is a hereditary condition in which normal hemoglobin is partly or completely replaced with abnormal hemoglobin S (Hgb S). Clinical manifestations occur primarily due to vaso-occlusion.
4. The thalassemias are a group of inherited blood disorders with anemia due to impaired hemoglobin synthesis. Clinical manifestations are usually detected in infancy, and include pallor, failure to thrive, hepatosplenomegaly, and severe anemia.

 SUGGESTION FOR CLASSROOM ACTIVITIES

- Demonstrate the concept of vaso-occlusion during sickle-cell disease with a piece of paper and an empty paper towel roll. Wad up the paper (normal RBC) into a tight ball and drop it through the paper towel roll (blood vessel). It passes through easily. Now shape the ball into a sickled cell, and note that it does not pass through the paper towel roll easily. Therefore, the distal tissues do not receive oxygen, leading to ischemic pain characteristic of the disease. You can also show the animation "Sickle Cell Anemia," available on *mynursingkit.com*

 SUGGESTION FOR CLINICAL ACTIVITIES

- It is common for the hospitalized child to have anemia. Discuss the possible reasons for a hospitalized child to become anemic. Have students identify iron-rich foods that children might eat.

LEARNING OUTCOME 3

Discuss the pathophysiology and clinical manifestations of the major disorders of white blood cells affecting the pediatric population.

Concepts for Lecture

1. Aplastic anemia is a failure of the bone marrow stem cells to produce all types of blood cells. Clinical manifestations are related to the degree of anemia, neutropenia, and thrombocytopenia that are present.

 POWERPOINT SLIDES 50–58

 VIDEO CLIPS

Nursing in Action: Administering Blood or Blood Products

 SUGGESTION FOR CLASSROOM ACTIVITIES

- Have students draw a concept map indicating how the clinical manifestations and laboratory findings of aplastic anemia are related to the pathophysiology of the disease process.

 SUGGESTION FOR CLINICAL ACTIVITIES

- Children with aplastic anemia often receive transfusions of blood products. Have students review this skill by watching the video "Administering Blood or Blood Products" activity, available on *mynursingkit.com*

LEARNING OUTCOME 4

Discuss the pathophysiology and clinical manifestations of the major bleeding disorders affecting the pediatric population.

Concepts for Lecture

1. Hemophilia, an X-linked recessive trait, is a group of disorders that occurs primarily in males and causes a deficiency of specific clotting factors. Clinical manifestations include mild to severe bleeding, bleeding into joint spaces, and bleeding from minor trauma.
2. Von Willebrand disease is a hereditary bleeding disorder that occurs in both men and women. Von Willebrand factor, which plays a necessary

 POWERPOINT SLIDES 59–75

 SUGGESTION FOR CLASSROOM ACTIVITIES

- Consider assigning Care Plan: "A School-Age Child with Hemophilia" available on *mynursingkit.com* before class and use it as a basis for discussion.

role in platelet adhesion, is deficient. Classic symptoms include easy bruising and epistaxis. Teenage girls may have menorrhagia.

3. Disseminated intravascular coagulation (DIC) is an acquired, abnormal activation of the clotting system that results in widespread clot formation throughout the body. After clotting factors have been used up, bleeding occurs. DIC is usually the result of other serious illnesses and common symptoms include bleeding and oozing, shock, and vessel thrombosis.

4. Idiopathic thrombocytopenic purpura (ITP) is a disorder where the spleen destroys the body's platelets. Platelet production in the bone marrow is normal. ITP is the most common bleeding disorder in children. Clinical manifestations include multiple bruises, petechiae, epistaxis, and blood in the urine or stool.

SUGGESTION FOR CLINICAL ACTIVITIES

- Monitor the operating room schedule; when a child is scheduled for splenectomy secondary to ITP, assign a student to observe the procedure.

LEARNING OUTCOME 5

Describe the nursing management and collaborative care of a child with a hematologic disorder.

Concepts for Lecture

1. The nursing management and collaborative care of hematologic disorders can be characterized in three groups: red blood cell disorders, white blood cell disorders, and clotting disorders.

2. Since hematologic disorders can be acute or chronic, there are a wide variety of medical and psychosocial issues that the family and child face. A team approach is the most effective method to support the family.

POWERPOINT SLIDES 76–80

VIDEO CLIPS

Nursing in Action: Administering Blood or Blood Products

SUGGESTION FOR CLASSROOM ACTIVITIES

- Before class, assign students to complete "Case Study: An Adolescent in Sickle Cell Crisis," available on *mynursingkit.com* as a basis for the discussion of the nursing care of a child with a hematologic disorder.

SUGGESTION FOR CLINICAL ACTIVITIES

- Invite the social worker or child life specialist from the hematology unit or clinic to talk to students during clinical conference about psychosocial support for families and children with hematologic disorders.

LEARNING OUTCOME 6

Discuss nursing implications for a child receiving hematopoietic stem cell transplantation (HSCT).

Concepts for Lecture

1. Hematopoietic stem cell transplantation (HSCT), also known as bone marrow transplantation, is a treatment used for diseases such as severe combined immunodeficiency syndrome, aplastic anemia, and leukemia. Stem cells exist primarily in the bone marrow but also circulate in the peripheral blood. There are three types of bone marrow transplant: autologous, isogeneic, and allogeneic.

2. Nursing management for the child with HSCT includes prevention of infection, controlling bleeding, maintaining adequate nutrition and hydration, monitoring for signs of rejection, and providing emotional support to the child and family.

POWERPOINT SLIDES 81–90

SUGGESTION FOR CLASSROOM ACTIVITIES

- Before class, assign students to research HSCT using the links provided in the Weblinks located on *mynursingkit.com*. Use their research findings as a framework for discussing this outcome.

SUGGESTIONS FOR CLINICAL ACTIVITIES

- If a bone marrow transplant unit is available in the local clinical setting, assign students to observe there.
- Review with students what is meant by "protective isolation," and how this type of isolation differs from traditional isolation.

GENERAL CHAPTER CONSIDERATIONS

1. Have students study and learn key terms listed at beginning of chapter.
2. Have students complete end-of-chapter exercises either in their book or on the MyNursingKit website.
3. Use the Classroom Response Questions provided in PowerPoint to assess students prior to lecture.

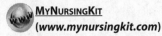

MYNURSINGKIT
(*www.mynursingkit.com*)

- NCLEX RN® review questions
- Case Studies
- Care Plans
- Critical Concept Review
- Thinking Critically
- Weblinks
- Weblink applications
- Nursing Tools
- Audio Glossary
- Images and Tables Library

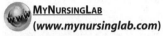

MYNURSINGLAB
(*www.mynursinglab.com*)

- Knowledge Quick Check
- Pre/Posttests
- Customized study plans
- Images and Tables Library
- *Separate purchase*

CLINICAL SKILLS MANUAL

- *Separate purchase*

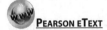

PEARSON ETEXT

- Students can search, highlight, take notes, and more all in electronic format
- *Separate purchase*

TESTBANK

CHAPTER 52
THE CHILD WITH CANCER

LEARNING OUTCOME 1

Describe the incidence, known etiologies, and common clinical manifestations of cancer.

Concepts for Lecture

1. In children under 15 years of age, cancer is the leading cause of disease-related death. However, mortality rates have improved and continue to improve. The overall survival rate for childhood cancer is 80%. Refer to Figure 52-1 to compare the most common forms of childhood cancers among children of different age groups.
2. The etiology of childhood cancer can be conceptually broken down into three categories: (1) external stimuli that cause genetic mutations, (2) immune system and gene abnormalities, and (3) chromosomal abnormalities.
3. Although some types of childhood cancer manifest no symptoms until the cancer is advanced, there may be several warning signs of childhood cancer. However, many of these symptoms are nonspecific, and are commonly seen with routine childhood illnesses.

 POWERPOINT SLIDES 19–25

Figure 52–1. Percentage of primary tumors by site of origin for different age groups

 VIDEO CLIPS

Cancer Overview

 SUGGESTIONS FOR CLASSROOM ACTIVITIES

- At the beginning of this class, show the video "Cancer Overview" (available on *mynursingkit.com*) as an introduction to the topic of childhood cancer.
- Using "Teaching Highlights: Ways to Decrease the Incidence of Cancer in Children," discuss actions nurses can take to educate children and families about the prevention of cancer.

 SUGGESTION FOR CLINICAL ACTIVITIES

- Determine the incidence of various types of childhood cancer in your local setting. Do the local patterns of cancer match the national patterns described in the text? Where do children go for treatment? What kinds of treatment are available locally?

LEARNING OUTCOME 2

Synthesize information about diagnostic tests and clinical therapy for cancer to plan comprehensive care for children undergoing these procedures.

Concepts for Lecture

1. Common diagnostic tests for childhood cancer include complete blood counts, bone marrow aspiration, lumbar puncture, imaging studies, and tumor biopsy. Refer to Table 52-1 for key points.
2. Clinical therapy for childhood cancer is complex. Cancer is treated with one or a combination of therapies, including surgery, chemotherapy, radiation, biotherapy, and bone marrow/stem-cell transplantation. The choice of treatment is determined by the type of cancer, its location, and the degree of metastasis.

 POWERPOINT SLIDES 26–40

Table 52–1. Selected diagnostic tests for childhood cancer

Table 52–2. Medications used for cancer chemotherapy

Feature Box: Pathophysiology Illustrated: Chemotherapy Drug Action

 SUGGESTIONS FOR CLASSROOM ACTIVITIES

- Use the information in "Pathophysiology Illustrated: Chemotherapy Drug Action," and Table 52-2 to discuss a sample chemotherapy treatment plan.
- Discuss the pros and cons of using umbilical blood as a source of stem cells.

SUGGESTIONS FOR CLINICAL ACTIVITIES

- Assign students to the pediatric imaging department to observe the diagnostic studies that may be used in diagnosing or treating childhood cancers.
- Discuss the difference in the automated versus manual differential of the complete blood count. Assign students to observe these laboratory analyses in the hospital laboratory.

LEARNING OUTCOME 3

Integrate information about oncologic emergencies into plans for monitoring all children with cancer.

Concepts for Lecture

1. Oncologic emergencies can be organized into three groups: metabolic, hematologic, and those involving space-occupying lesions.
2. Metabolic emergencies result from the lysis of tumor cells, a process called tumor lysis syndrome. Septic shock and hypercalcemia are also considered metabolic emergencies.
3. Hematologic emergencies result from bone marrow suppression or hyperleukocytosis.
4. Space-occupying lesions occur when rapid tumor growth causes compression, resulting in increased pressure or obstruction.

POWERPOINT SLIDES 41–48

SUGGESTION FOR CLASSROOM ACTIVITIES

- To illustrate the concept of space-occupying lesions, bring a balloon and a cardboard box to class. Cut a small hole in the cardboard box and place the end of balloon through the hole. As you blow up the balloon, explain that the balloon represents the rapidly expanding tumor growth, which can then compress surrounding tissue (as in the spinal cord or superior vena cava) or increase pressure (as in intracranial pressure).

SUGGESTION FOR CLINICAL ACTIVITIES

- Assign students to the pediatric oncology unit and have them discuss the management of hematologic emergencies with nurses who work on the unit.

LEARNING OUTCOME 4

Recognize the most common solid tumors in children, describe their treatment, and plan comprehensive nursing care.

Concepts for Lecture

1. Brain tumors are the most common solid tumors in children. The cause of most brain tumors is unknown. These tumors manifest by behavioral or nervous system changes that occur either rapidly or more slowly and subtly. Although treatment varies with the type of tumor, surgery, radiation, and chemotherapy are typically used. Nursing management focuses on coordination of care, postoperative care, administering medications, and monitoring for complications.
2. Neuroblastoma is a smooth, hard, nontender mass that can occur anywhere along the sympathetic nervous system chain. Common locations include the abdominal, adrenal, thoracic, and cervical areas. Clinical manifestations depend upon the location of the mass. Surgery, followed by chemotherapy, is usually the therapy of choice. Nursing management includes postoperative care, medication administration, and teaching.
3. Wilms' tumor (also known as nephroblastoma) is a common intrarenal tumor that accounts for 6% of all childhood tumors. The tumor is usually asymptomatic, although a mass may be present. Therapy involves surgery and chemotherapy or radiation therapy. Nursing management focuses on postoperative care and chemotherapy monitoring and administration.

POWERPOINT SLIDES 49–70

Feature Box: Pathophysiology Illustrated: Brain Tumors

SUGGESTION FOR CLASSROOM ACTIVITIES

- Before class, assign students to review the "Case Study: A Child with Cancer" located on *mynursingkit.com*. In class, change the patient to a teen with Ewing's sarcoma. Use the case study as a basis for discussion about nursing management of adolescents with bone tumors.

SUGGESTION FOR CLINICAL ACTIVITIES

- Find out if a support group exists locally for children who have had limbs amputated. If it does, assign students to attend the group. If it does not exist, students could help facilitate such a group.

4. Bone tumors include osteosarcoma and Ewing's sarcoma. Osteosarcoma is the most common skeletal tumor in children, and is primarily seen during the adolescent growth spurt. Osteosarcoma is most commonly seen in the femur, tibia, or humerus. Ewing's sarcoma is a small malignant tumor that involves the shaft of the long bones. Clinical manifestations include pain, swelling, and some laboratory abnormalities. Nursing management includes postoperative care and monitoring. Children who have had limbs amputated often have concerns regarding body image.

LEARNING OUTCOME 5

Plan care for children and adolescents of all ages who have a diagnosis of leukemia.

Concepts for Lecture

1. Leukemia, characterized by an abnormal proliferation of white blood cells, is the most common form of pediatric cancer. The two most common forms of leukemia are acute lymphoblastic leukemia (ALL) and acute nonlymphocytic leukemia (also known as acute myelogenous leukemia [AML]).
2. The pathophysiology of leukemia involves a large number of immature white blood cells that replace normal white blood cells. This leaves the body vulnerable to infection, and eventually results in anemia and thrombocytopenia.
3. Clinical manifestations are directly related to the pathophysiology of the disease process. In addition, symptoms may be related to infiltration and the resulting mass and pressure effect.
4. Leukemia is diagnosed based on blood counts and bone marrow aspiration. Therapy involves radiation and chemotherapy. The most important prognostic indicator is the initial leukocyte count: The higher it is upon a diagnosis, the worse the prognosis.
5. Nursing management focuses on assessment, diagnosis, planning and implementation, and evaluation.

LEARNING OUTCOME 6

Recognize the most common soft-tissue tumors in children, describe their treatment, and plan comprehensive care.

Concepts for Lecture

1. Soft-tissue tumors include Hodgkin disease, non-Hodgkin lymphoma, rhabdomyosarcoma, and retinoblastoma.
2. Hodgkin disease is a disorder of the lymphoid system that occurs most commonly in adolescent boys. The main symptom is a nontender, firm lymph node that is usually in the supraclavicular or cervical nodes. After diagnosis via lymph node biopsy, therapy includes chemotherapy and radiation.
3. Non-Hodgkin lymphoma is a malignant tumor of the lymphoreticular system. It is the third most common group of malignancies in children (following leukemia and brain tumors). Children usually present with fever and weight loss, as well as enlarged lymph nodes. Chemotherapy is the primary form of therapy.
4. Rhabdomyosarcoma occurs most often in the muscles of the eyes and neck, although it can occur in other muscles as well. Clinical

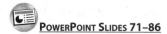

POWERPOINT SLIDES 71–86

Feature Box: Nursing Practice: Laboratory Values in Leukemia

VIDEO CLIPS

Leukemia

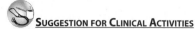

SUGGESTION FOR CLASSROOM ACTIVITIES

- At the beginning of this portion of the class, show the video "Leukemia," located on *mynursingkit.com*. Use this video as an introduction to this topic.

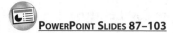

SUGGESTION FOR CLINICAL ACTIVITIES

- Ask a child and family with leukemia to talk with students during a clinical conference about what it is like to live with the disease and what hospitalizations are like.

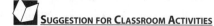

POWERPOINT SLIDES 87–103

Figure 52–10. Rhabdomyosarcoma

Figure 52–11. Retinoblastoma

Feature Box: Pathophysiology Illustrated: Hodgkin Disease

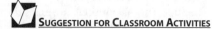

SUGGESTION FOR CLASSROOM ACTIVITIES

- Divide students into groups and have each group draw (on an overhead transparency or a large piece of paper from a flip chart) a basic sketch of a child with one of the soft-tissue tumors described above. They should include depictions of each clinical manifestation on their sketch. Have the rest of the class guess which disease process has been drawn and use this activity as the basis for discussing the rest of the outcome.

manifestations vary based on the tumor site. The tumor is removed via surgery, and therapy then focuses on chemotherapy and radiation.

5. Retinoblastoma is an intraocular malignancy of the retina that may be bilateral or unilateral. A white pupil (leukokoria) is the main clinical sign. Radiation, chemotherapy, and surgery are all typical therapies, and the eye may be surgically removed.

Learning Outcome 7

Describe the impact of cancer survival on children and use this information to plan for ongoing physiologic and psychosocial care in the children's futures.

Concepts for Lecture

1. The diagnosis of "cancer" can be devastating, and children often react differently to the diagnosis than their parents do.
2. Psychosocial assessment focuses on body image, stress and coping abilities, support systems, and developmental level.
3. There can be many long-term physiologic effects of therapies used to treat cancer.

General Chapter Considerations

1. Have students study and learn key terms listed at beginning of chapter.
2. Have students complete end-of-chapter exercises either in their book or on the MyNursingKit website.
3. Use the Classroom Response Questions provided in PowerPoint to assess students prior to lecture.

SUGGESTION FOR CLINICAL ACTIVITIES

- Assign students to observe in an outpatient pediatric chemotherapy clinic. Students should have the opportunity to interact with many children with soft-tissue tumors.

POWERPOINT SLIDES 104–111

SUGGESTION FOR CLASSROOM ACTIVITIES

- Invite a social worker, case manager, or child life specialist who works with children and families with cancer to speak to the class about the effects the cancer diagnosis has on families.

SUGGESTION FOR CLINICAL ACTIVITIES

- Students are often hesitant to assess and plan interventions in the psychosocial realm. When caring for these children, have students write three age-appropriate questions that they can use with the child and his or her family to encourage discussion about psychosocial issues.

MyNursingKit
(www.mynursingkit.com)

- NCLEX RN® review questions
- Case Studies
- Care Plans
- Critical Concept Review
- Thinking Critically
- Weblinks
- Weblink applications
- Nursing Tools
- Audio Glossary
- Images and Tables Library

MyNursingLab
(www.mynursinglab.com)

- Knowledge Quick Check
- Pre/Posttests
- Customized study plans
- Images and Tables Library
- *Separate purchase*

CLINICAL SKILLS MANUAL

- *Separate purchase*

PEARSON eTEXT

- Students can search, highlight, take notes, and more all in electronic format
- *Separate purchase*

TESTBANK

CHAPTER 53
THE CHILD WITH ALTERATIONS IN GASTROINTESTINAL FUNCTION

LEARNING OUTCOME 1

Describe the general function of the gastrointestinal system.

Concepts for Lecture

1. General functions of the gastrointestinal system include ingestion, digestion, and absorption of fluids and nutrients; metabolism of needed nutrients; and excretion of waste products.
2. The gastrointestinal tract, while structurally complete at birth, undergoes changes as the infant grows and develops in order to make it functionally mature.

 POWERPOINT SLIDES 19–24

 ANIMATION

Digestive System

 SUGGESTION FOR CLASSROOM ACTIVITIES

- As an introduction to this topic, show the animation "Digestive System," available on *mynursingkit.com*

 SUGGESTION FOR CLINICAL ACTIVITIES

- Ask students how they would explain the basic functions of the gastrointestinal tract to children of various ages. They can use these concepts when they teach children and families during their clinical rotations.

LEARNING OUTCOME 2

Discuss the pathophysiological processes associated with specific gastrointestinal disorders in the pediatric population.

Concepts for Lecture

1. Structural defects occur when the growth and development of fetal structures are interrupted during the first trimester. Examples of structural defects include cleft lip and palate, esophageal atresia with tracheoesophageal fistula, and pyloric stenosis.
2. Intussusception is one of the most frequent causes of intestinal obstruction in infancy and occurs when one portion of the intestine prolapses and telescopes into itself.
3. The two major abdominal wall defects common in children include omphalocele and gastroschisis. Omphalocele tends to be associated with other congenital anomalies, while gastroschisis tends to be an isolated defect.
4. Anorectal malformations are common congenital anomalies and can range from minor to complex. Anorectal malformations may occur in isolation or may be associated with other congenial defects.
5. A hernia is a protrusion of an organ or part of an organ through the muscle wall of the cavity that normally contains it. Diaphragmatic hernia and umbilical hernia are two types of hernias seen in children, although inguinal hernias are the most common. (Note: Inguinal hernias are covered in Chapter 54.)
6. Gastroesophageal reflux (GER), Hirschsprung disease, gastroenteritis, constipation, and encopresis are disorders of motility. GER affects about half of all children, although only a small portion will go on to develop gastroesophageal reflux disease.

 POWERPOINT SLIDES 25–76

Figure 53–1A. Cleft lip. *A,* Unilateral cleft lip

Figure 53–1B. Cleft lip. *B,* Bilateral cleft lip

Figure 53–3. Omphalocele

Figure 53–4. Gastroschisis

Figure 53–6. Umbilical hernia

Figure 53–8. Celiac disease

Feature Box: Clinical Manifestations: Common Intestinal Parasitic Disorders

 VIDEO CLIPS

Nursing in Action: Ostomy Care

 VIDEO CLIPS

Stool Toileting: Refusals and Rewards

7. Volvulus, also known as malrotation, occurs when the bowel fails to rotate counterclockwise into its permanent position in the intestine. The result is disruption of bloodflow and necrosis of the intestine.
8. Many underlying conditions can necessitate ostomy placement in the pediatric population.
9. Inflammatory disorders are reactions of specific tissues of the GI tract to trauma caused by injuries, foreign bodies, chemicals, microorganisms, or surgery. Disorders in this category include appendicitis, peptic ulcers, necrotizing enterocolitis, Meckel's diverticulum, and inflammatory bowel disease.
10. Celiac disease, lactose intolerance, and short bowel syndrome represent three types of malabsorption disorders, defined by the lack of digestion or absorption of nutrients.
11. Colic and rumination are two types of feeding disorders that are common in infants and young children.
12. Hepatic disorders include biliary atresia and hepatitis. Cirrhosis of the liver may also occur. Children most likely to get hepatitis A or hepatitis B. Biliary atresia is the most common pediatric liver disease necessitating transplant.
13. Children can contract many parasitic diseases that affect the gastrointestinal tract. See Clinical Manifestations: "Common Intestinal Parasitic Disorders" for a complete discussion of these diseases.

LEARNING OUTCOME 3

Identify signs and symptoms that may indicate a disorder of the gastrointestinal system.

Concepts for Lecture

1. Signs and symptoms of gastrointestinal illnesses tend to be nonspecific and overlap from disease to disease.

LEARNING OUTCOME 4

Contrast nursing management and plan care for disorders of the gastrointestinal system for the child needing abdominal surgery versus the child needing nonoperative management.

Concepts for Lecture

1. There are several components of general nursing care that should be done for any child with a gastrointestinal disorder.

 SUGGESTION FOR CLASSROOM ACTIVITIES

- Use a long, cylindrical balloon to illustrate the pathophysiology of intussusception. After the balloon is lightly inflated, use your finger to push one end of it into the lumen, mimicking what happens in the intestine during intussusception.

 SUGGESTION FOR CLINICAL ACTIVITIES

- Many gastrointestinal disorders in childhood are treated surgically. When possible, assign students to observe in the pediatric operating room the surgical correction and treatment of these disorders.

 POWERPOINT SLIDES 77–79

 SUGGESTIONS FOR CLASSROOM ACTIVITIES

- For each gastrointestinal disease described in the chapter, have students make a list of signs and symptoms that are different from the general symptoms described previously. This list can help them learn how to differentiate these diseases.
- Bring a jar of currant jelly purchased from a grocery store to illustrate the type of stools that may be seen in children with intussusception.

 SUGGESTION FOR CLINICAL ACTIVITIES

- Demonstrate how to perform an abdominal exam on children of different ages. For example, students often have difficulty performing exams on infants and toddlers who cannot describe symptoms of pain. Strategies and tips for assessing young children can be discussed.

 POWERPOINT SLIDES 80–91

 SUGGESTION FOR CLASSROOM ACTIVITIES

- Before class, assign students to complete "Care Plan: The Child with Cleft Palate," available on *mynursingkit.com*. Use this case as a basis for discussing the nursing care of children with this disorder.

2. Nursing management of common gastrointestinal disorders includes the general principles described previously, as well as actions specific to each surgical and nonsurgical disease process.

LEARNING OUTCOME 5

Analyze developmentally appropriate approaches for nursing management of gastrointestinal disorders in the pediatric population.

Concepts for Lecture

1. The principles of growth and development should be applied in the nursing management of children across the lifespan with gastrointestinal disorders.

LEARNING OUTCOME 6

Discuss nursing management of the child with an injury to the abdomen.

Concepts for Lecture

1. In children, the majority of abdominal trauma is blunt trauma sustained in motor vehicle crashes, auto-pedestrian accidents, and abuse. Nursing care focuses on monitoring the child's status, as well as providing interventions as needed.

 SUGGESTION FOR CLINICAL ACTIVITIES
- Assign students to observe in a pediatric outpatient gastrointestinal clinic to gain exposure to how these disorders are monitored and treated throughout the child's life.

 POWERPOINT SLIDES 92–96

 SUGGESTION FOR CLASSROOM ACTIVITIES
- Divide the class to represent the four age groups (infant, toddler, child, adolescent). Give them a handout with three gastrointestinal disorders that span a lifetime. Have each group decide what would be the appropriate nursing care based on each age group. Tell them to include play, safety, education, and nursing interaction.

 SUGGESTION FOR CLINICAL ACTIVITIES
- Assign students to shadow a dietitian in order to learn how to address the dietary aspects of pediatric gastrointestinal disorders.

 POWERPOINT SLIDES 97–100

 SUGGESTION FOR CLASSROOM ACTIVITIES
- Compare management of splenic trauma in the pediatric population to the adult population. Why is there an emphasis on salvaging spleens in children? Have students consider the role of the spleen in immune function when thinking about this question.

 SUGGESTION FOR CLINICAL ACTIVITIES
- Assign students to observe in the pediatric emergency room, and discuss the role of the emergency room staff when a child presents with abdominal trauma.

GENERAL CHAPTER CONSIDERATIONS

1. Have students study and learn key terms listed at beginning of chapter.
2. Have students complete end-of-chapter exercises either in their book or on the MyNursingKit website.
3. Use the Classroom Response Questions provided in PowerPoint to assess students prior to lecture.

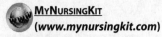

MyNursingKit
(*www.mynursingkit.com*)

- NCLEX RN® review questions
- Case Studies
- Care Plans
- Critical Concept Review
- Thinking Critically
- Weblinks
- Weblink applications
- Nursing Tools
- Audio Glossary
- Images and Tables Library

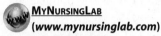

MyNursingLab
(*www.mynursinglab.com*)

- Knowledge Quick Check
- Pre/Posttests
- Customized study plans
- Images and Tables Library
- *Separate purchase*

CLINICAL SKILLS MANUAL

- *Separate purchase*

PEARSON eTEXT

- Students can search, highlight, take notes, and more all in electronic format
- *Separate purchase*

TESTBANK

CHAPTER 54
THE CHILD WITH ALTERATIONS IN GENITOURINARY FUNCTION

LEARNING OUTCOME 1

Describe the pathophysiologic processes associated with genitourinary disorders in the pediatric population.

Concepts for Lecture

1. Enuresis is repeated involuntary voiding by a child old enough that bladder control is expected, usually about 5 to 6 years of age. Enuresis can result from neurologic or congenital structural disorders, illness, or stress. Treatment includes bladder training, fluid restriction, enuresis alarms, and medication. See "Nursing Practice: Questions to Ask When Taking an Enuresis History" and Table 54-3: "Treatment Approaches for Enuresis."

2. Nephrotic syndrome is a clinical state characterized by edema, massive proteinuria, hypoalbuminemia, hypoproteinemia, hyperlipidemia, and altered immunity. Generalized edema of the extremities, abdomen, and genitals usually prompts parents to seek treatment, which includes steroids, albumin, and diuretics. Refer to "Drug Guide: Prednisone" for details.

3. Renal failure is classified as acute or chronic. Acute renal failure usually occurs suddenly (days to weeks) and may be reversible, where chronic renal failure occurs over months to years and is usually not reversible. Diagnostic tests and clinical manifestations between the two vary. Hyperkalemia is the most life-threatening complication of renal failure.

4. Polycystic kidney disease (PKD) is a genetic disorder where cystic sacs form in the collecting ducts of the kidneys. Eventually, urinary flow is obstructed. Severe forms of PKD may cause renal failure shortly after birth, whereas less severe forms of PKD may not cause symptoms until later in the child's life.

5. Hemolytic-uremic syndrome (HUS) is an acute renal disease characterized by hemolytic anemia, thrombocytopenia, and acute renal failure. The most common cause is a toxin produced by *E. coli* 0157:H7 that is often found in undercooked ground beef. Most children recover from the disease, but some may go on to develop chronic renal failure.

6. Acute postinfectious glomerulonephritis (APIGN) is an inflammation of the glomeruli of the kidneys, and is triggered by deposition of antigen-antibody complexes in the glomeruli. The most common organism that triggers this response is Group A streptococcal infections of the skin and pharynx. Treatment is symptomatic, and most children recover within a few weeks.

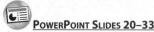 **POWERPOINT SLIDES 20–33**

Feature Box: Pathophysiology Illustrated: Nephrotic Syndrome

Table 54-3. Treatment approaches for enuresis

Table 54-4. Diagnostic tests for renal failure

 ANIMATION
Renal Function

ANIMATION
Furosemide

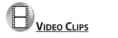 **VIDEO CLIPS**
Sexually Transmitted Infections

SUGGESTIONS FOR CLASSROOM ACTIVITIES

- Before class, create a list of assessment data and laboratory values typical for a client with one of the renal disorders described previously. Challenge the students to analyze the data and determine which disease the client has. By creating several different scenarios, students can learn to differentiate these disorders. (Hint: refer to Table 54-4, "Diagnostic Tests for Renal Failure" to help students during this exercise.)

- Furosemide is a common diuretic used in several of the previously mentioned conditions. Show the animation "Furosemide," available on *mynursingkit.com*. Ask students to identify why hypokalemia is a common side effect of furosemide. Discussion about the onset of action, duration, and monitoring of the client on diuretics is also appropriate

- When discussing acute postinfectious glomerulonephritis (APIGN) during lecture, show the animation "Renal Function" available on *mynursingkit.com*. This brief animation shows students exactly where the glomeruli are located, and you can point out that the antigen-antibody complexes that "clog up" the glomeruli are carried through the blood.

LEARNING OUTCOME 2

Discuss the nursing management of a child with a structural defect of the genitourinary system.

Concepts for Lecture

1. Bladder exstrophy occurs when the posterior bladder wall extrudes through the lower abdominal wall. Preoperative nursing care includes prevention of infection and trauma to the exposed bladder. Post-op care includes immobilization to promote pelvic closure, wound care, pain control, and monitoring of renal function.

2. Hypospadias and epispadias are congenital anomalies involving the abnormal location of the urethral meatus in males. After surgical repair, nursing priorities include pain management, monitoring urine output, and monitoring of the urinary stent (if present).

3. Obstructive uropathies—congenital abnormalities that interfere with urine flow—include ureteropelvic junction (UPJ) obstruction and posterior urethral valves. Prune-belly syndrome is a congenital defect in which the abdominal musculature does not develop. The end result of these defects is hydronephrosis, which leads to renal failure if left untreated.

4. Phimosis occurs when the foreskin over the glans penis cannot be pulled back, usually due to infection or adhesions. Treatment includes betamethasone cream or circumcision.

5. Cryptorchidism (undescended testes) occurs when one or both testes fail to descend through the inguinal canal into the scrotum. Surgical correction is carried out by 1 year of age to prevent complications of uncorrected cryptorchidism, which include infertility and malignancy. Surgery is usually done on an outpatient basis, and discharge teaching is a nursing priority.

6. Inguinal hernia occurs when abdominal tissue—usually bowel—extends into the inguinal canal. Incarceration describes a hernia that cannot be reduced and has impaired circulation, which is a medical emergency. Surgical correction is usually an outpatient procedure, and nursing management involves discharge teaching, pain control, and wound care.

7. Testicular torsion is an emergency condition in which the testis suddenly rotates on its spermatic cord, cutting off its blood supply. Surgery must be done within 4 to 6 hours in order to restore blood supply to the testis. Since the child often goes home within a few hours of the surgery, nursing care is focused on discharge teaching.

POWERPOINT SLIDES 34–46

Figure 54–2. Bladder exstrophy

Figure 54–3. Hypospadias and epispadias

Feature Box: Pathophysiology Illustrated: Obstruction Sites in the Urinary System

VIDEO CLIPS

Circumcision

SUGGESTIONS FOR CLASSROOM ACTIVITIES

• After discussing phimosis, show the video "Circumcision" on *mynursingkit.com*. The video discusses the purpose of circumcision, as well as cultural and geographic variations in the practice. After viewing the video, have students discuss factors that families might consider in deciding whether or not to circumcise a newborn baby boy.

• Ask students to pretend that they are working in a clinic when a 12-year-old boy arrives vomiting and with abdominal pain. During his intake interview, he reveals to the nurse that he is also having pain "down there." The pain started about 4 or 5 hours ago, but he was too embarrassed to tell his mother. The nurse suspects that he may have testicular torsion. Have students role-play how they would deal with this client. Key points include providing privacy during the examination, thorough assessment, and urgent referral to the emergency department. The client may have questions about fertility and the surgical procedure to correct testicular torsion that can be worked into the scenario.

SUGGESTION FOR CLINICAL ACTIVITIES

• When a student is caring for a patient who has had urological surgery, have the student draw the urinary system before and after the surgery. Include any drains, stents, or catheters that are present. Discuss the purpose of each of these tubes, as well as the expected output from each tube. Many students are visual learners, and drawing this "map" of their client can increase their understanding of both the pathophysiology and the treatment.

LEARNING OUTCOME 3

Develop a nursing care plan for the child with a urinary tract infection.

Concepts for Lecture

1. Urinary tract infections (UTIs) can either be acute or chronic and can occur anywhere along the urinary tract. This includes the upper urinary tract (pyelonephritis involving the kidneys and ureters) and lower urinary tract (cystitis involving the bladder and/or urethra).
2. UTIs are very common in children. Males have higher rates of structural defects of the urinary tract, leading to higher rates in males versus females during the newborn and infancy stage. Girls have higher rates after infancy due to the shorter female urethra and its proximity to the anus, which increases exposure to fecal bacteria.
3. Most UTIs are caused by *E. coli,* especially if this is the child's first UTI. Other causative agents are possible.
4. Symptoms of UTI in newborns are nonspecific, including fever, failure to thrive, poor feeding, vomiting and diarrhea, strong-smelling urine, and irritability. After the toddler years, symptoms of UTIs are similar to those of adults. Many UTIs are asymptomatic. Refer to "Teaching Highlights: Prevention of Urinary Tract Infections."
5. Antibiotics are the treatment of choice. Follow-up cultures should be sterile.

LEARNING OUTCOME 4

Discuss the growth and developmental issues for the child with chronic renal failure.

Concepts for Lecture

1. Children with chronic renal failure often have delayed physical growth and maturation due to the effects of uremia on hormones. Puberty is often delayed.
2. While chronic renal failure in and of itself is not associated with developmental delays, children with the disease may have difficulty with social adjustment and success in school. Screening the younger child with appropriate developmental screening tests, such as the Denver II, should be a part of the child's assessment.
3. Chronic renal failure presents many challenges for the child and family, including coping with altered body image, short stature, delayed onset of puberty, and possible physical side effects of medications. If the child is receiving hemodialysis, he or she may miss significant time in school.

 POWERPOINT SLIDES 47–52

 SUGGESTION FOR CLASSROOM ACTIVITIES

- Divide students into groups of 4 to 6 and have each group develop the nursing care plan for a child with a UTI. Have them write their answers on an overhead transparency. Compare the various care plans and discuss differences among the various groups. In addition to correcting errors or omissions, this activity allows students to see the variations in how nursing care is prioritized.

 SUGGESTION FOR CLINICAL ACTIVITIES

- Discuss various methods for obtaining urine specimens in children of different ages (infants, toddlers, school age, adolescents). Encourage students to review "Skill 16-1: Performing a Urinary Catheterization" in the *Clinical Skills Manual.* Discuss the differences in catheterizing children versus adults.

 POWERPOINT SLIDES 53–58

 SUGGESTIONS FOR CLASSROOM ACTIVITIES

- Invite a family who has a child with chronic renal failure to attend your class. Have students prepare one or two questions to ask the family. Allow the parents and the child (if age is appropriate) to share the child's story regarding renal failure and dialysis. The family will likely discuss many of the concepts in this outcome.
- Divide students into groups of 4 to 6 people. Have each group read "Evidence-Based Nursing: Living with End-Stage Renal Disease," then have each group list three things they would consider in the future when working with children and families coping with ESRD.

 SUGGESTION FOR CLINICAL ACTIVITIES

- When taking care of a child or adolescent with chronic renal failure, discuss the concept of nonadherence with the student. Novice students often assume that all clients adhere to the prescribed treatment, and students may become judgmental when this does not occur. If nonadherence was the reason for admission (e.g., missed dialysis treatments, not taking medications, etc.), discuss strategies that the nurse can use to improve adherence.

LEARNING OUTCOME 5

Summarize dietary restrictions for the child with a renal disorder.

Concepts for Lecture

1. The type of diet prescribed for the child depends on the pathophysiology of the renal disorder.
2. Growth in children with renal disorders is important, and most diets include high amounts of calories and protein. The protein intake must be balanced with the azotemia, as BUN and creatinine will rise with high protein intake.
3. In the presence of renal failure, sodium, potassium, and phosphorus are often restricted. Normal, healthy kidneys control sodium balance through fluid balance, and remove excess potassium and phosphorus from the body through the urine. During renal failure, these three electrolytes tend to accumulate.
4. The renal dietitian is a powerful ally for the nurse who is caring for a child with a renal disorder.

LEARNING OUTCOME 6

Develop a nursing care plan for the child with acute and chronic renal failure on dialysis.

Concepts for Lecture

1. Although there are differences, acute and chronic renal failure have many parallels regarding nursing care. Families who have children being treated with peritoneal dialysis at home have significant educational needs.

 POWERPOINT SLIDES 59–67

Table 54–5. Nutritional information for the child with kidney disease

 SUGGESTION FOR CLASSROOM ACTIVITIES

- Divide students into groups of 4 to 6 people. Ask them to make a list of the foods they ate the day before. Have them refer to Table 54-5. Have them cross through any foods that they could not eat if they were on a diet that restricted sodium, potassium, and phosphorus. Students will discover that the electrolyte-restricted diet is very bland and extremely difficult to follow. This can give them insight into the challenges these clients face.

 SUGGESTION FOR CLINICAL ACTIVITIES

- Have students explore the clinical setting for resources regarding the renal diet. For example, if they had a patient who was on a low-sodium, low-potassium, and low-phosphorus diet, how would they evaluate the food tray before taking it into the patient's room? Resources regarding foods high in these electrolytes can be found in many places in the clinical setting: textbooks, client education materials, the dietary office, the World Wide Web, and the dialysis clinic.

 POWERPOINT SLIDES 68–74

Feature Box: Clinical Manifestations: Acute Versus Chronic Renal Failure

Feature Box: Developing Cultural Competence: Reducing Sodium in the Child's Diet

 SUGGESTION FOR CLASSROOM ACTIVITIES

- Ask the students to refer to "Developing Cultural Competence: Reducing Sodium in the Child's Diet." Identify unique characteristics of the diet of cultures present in your community that may present challenges for the child with renal failure. For example, the Hispanic diet often includes cheese, tomatoes, and beef—all of which could be restricted due to electrolyte content. If time allows, students can then propose alternatives that could be suggested to clients.
- Assign "Care Plan: A Child with Nephrotic Syndrome" activity available on *mynursingkit.com* for review.

- When students are caring for a child with chronic renal failure, ask them to draw a concept map to relate the pathophysiology of the disease with the medications and the labs. For example, students can visually relate the following points: During renal failure, the kidneys do not produce erythropoietin, which leads to anemia. This is treated with synthetic erythropoietin, which is monitored by the hemoglobin and hematocrit, as well as the reticulocyte count. Since chronic renal failure is a disease with complex pathophysiology, multiple medications, and numerous labs, the concept map can help students make connections that might otherwise be overlooked.

Learning Outcome 7

Describe psychosocial issues for the child requiring surgery on the genitourinary system.

Concepts for Lecture

1. Infants who have had genitourinary surgery may have issues with bonding and trust if their basic needs are not met.
2. Toddlers and school-age children who have had genitourinary surgery may not achieve urinary continence. This can lead to issues with self-esteem and self-confidence.
3. Adolescents who have had genitourinary surgery may also have issues with self-esteem and self-confidence. They may have difficulty achieving sexual identity and may have concerns about fertility and sexual function. Children who have uncomplicated genitourinary surgery or who have no loss of function or continence are less likely to have psychosocial issues than children who have complicated repairs with residual defects.

POWERPOINT SLIDES 75–78

SUGGESTION FOR CLASSROOM ACTIVITIES

- Have students role-play how they would approach children with the preceding psychosocial issues. For infants and toddlers, one student can be the parent and the other can be the nurse. For adolescents, one student can be the adolescent and the other can be the nurse. Teaching points include close attention to body language, asking open-ended questions, and developing a trusting therapeutic relationship.

SUGGESTION FOR CLINICAL ACTIVITIES

- Have students consult with a child life specialist in the clinical setting. Ask the student to make a list of three strategies for dealing with psychosocial issues in each age group. These can be shared during clinical conference.

GENERAL CHAPTER CONSIDERATIONS

1. Have students study and learn key terms listed at beginning of chapter.
2. Have students complete end-of-chapter exercises either in their book or on the MyNursingKit website.
3. Use the Classroom Response Questions provided in PowerPoint to assess students prior to lecture.

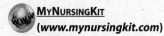

MYNURSINGKIT
(*www.mynursingkit.com*)

- NCLEX RN® review questions
- Case Studies
- Care Plans
- Critical Concept Review
- Thinking Critically
- Weblinks
- Weblink applications
- Nursing Tools
- Audio Glossary
- Images and Tables Library

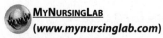

MYNURSINGLAB
(*www.mynursinglab.com*)

- Knowledge Quick Check
- Pre/Posttests
- Customized study plans
- Images and Tables Library
- *Separate purchase*

CLINICAL SKILLS MANUAL

- *Separate purchase*

PEARSON ETEXT

- Students can search, highlight, take notes, and more all in electronic format
- *Separate purchase*

TESTBANK

CHAPTER 55
THE CHILD WITH ALTERATIONS IN ENDOCRINE FUNCTION

LEARNING OUTCOME 1

Identify the function of important hormones of the endocrine system.

Concepts for Lecture

1. The endocrine system controls the cellular activity that regulates growth and metabolism. Hormones are chemical messengers in the body. Several important hormones are reviewed in the text, including gonadotropin-releasing hormone, growth hormone, antidiuretic hormone, thyroid and parathyroid hormones, and insulin. Table 55-1 provides an overview of additional hormones in the body.

POWERPOINT SLIDES 19–23

Table 55–1. Endocrine glands and their functions

ANIMATION

Endocrine System: Secretion of Hormones

SUGGESTION FOR CLASSROOM ACTIVITIES

- When introducing the endocrine system, use the animation "Endocrine System: Secretion of Hormones," available on *mynursingkit.com* to illustrate the physiology of the endocrine system.

SUGGESTION FOR CLINICAL ACTIVITIES

- When students are caring for a child with an endocrine dysfunction, have the student draw the regulatory pathway for that hormone. This exercise will help the student understand the pathophysiology of the disease, as well as diagnostic tests, signs and symptoms, and medications used to treat the disease.

LEARNING OUTCOME 2

Identify signs and symptoms that may indicate a disorder of the endocrine system.

Concepts for Lecture

1. There are general "red flags" that may indicate a disorder of the endocrine system. These symptoms can be grouped into categories that include growth, metabolism, mental retardation, sexual development, changes in urine output or thirst, and Cushingoid features.

POWERPOINT SLIDES 24–31

SUGGESTION FOR CLASSROOM ACTIVITIES

- Before class, assign students to complete the activity "Weblink Applications: A Child with Turner's Syndrome," available on *mynursingkit.com*

SUGGESTION FOR CLINICAL ACTIVITIES

- Invite a pediatric endocrinologist to speak to the group during a clinical conference and ask him or her to discuss ways that nurses can identify children at risk for endocrine disorders.

LEARNING OUTCOME 3

Identify all conditions for which short stature is a sign.

Concepts for Lecture

1. Numerous disorders have short stature as a finding. For this reason, it is important for nurses to know how to plot a child's height on a growth chart.

POWERPOINT SLIDES 32–34

SUGGESTION FOR CLASSROOM ACTIVITIES

- Based on their knowledge of pathophysiology, challenge the class to explain why short stature is a sign of the conditions discussed in this outcome.

SUGGESTION FOR CLINICAL ACTIVITIES

- During clinical time, have students measure the height of various children and plot the results on a growth chart.

LEARNING OUTCOME 4

Develop a nursing care plan for each type of acquired metabolic disorder.

Concepts for Lecture

1. The nursing care of children with acquired metabolic disorders includes teaching children and families about the disorder, administering medications, and carrying out diagnostic tests. Some children are at risk for fluid and electrolyte imbalances and require monitoring, dietary changes, and fluid and electrolyte replacement. Children who have alterations in body image may need support to develop a positive self-image.

POWERPOINT SLIDES 35–43

SUGGESTION FOR CLASSROOM ACTIVITIES

- Divide the class into groups and have each group briefly present the disorder and associated nursing care to the class.

SUGGESTION FOR CLINICAL ACTIVITIES

- Assign students to post-op units where many children with these disorders are cared for after surgery.

LEARNING OUTCOME 5

Develop a family education plan for the child that needs lifelong cortisol replacement.

Concepts for Lecture

1. Families with children who require lifelong cortisol replacement need education about medication administration, as well as knowledge of the symptoms of acute adrenal insufficiency.

POWERPOINT SLIDES 44–48

SUGGESTION FOR CLASSROOM ACTIVITIES

- Challenge students to explain the pathophysiology of the signs of adrenal insufficiency.

SUGGESTION FOR CLINICAL ACTIVITIES

- Have students determine what teaching materials are available in the local clinical setting to use with children and families who require lifelong cortisol replacement.

LEARNING OUTCOME 6

Distinguish between the nursing care of the child with type 1 and type 2 diabetes.

Concepts for Lecture

1. Nursing care of the child with type 1 diabetes focuses on monitoring blood glucose, education, medication administration, and teaching.

POWERPOINT SLIDES 49–55

ANIMATION

Physiology of Diabetes

The family also needs to understand the underlying pathophysiology of the condition.

2. Nursing care of the child with type 2 diabetes includes monitoring blood glucose, education, and teaching. Medications usually include oral hypoglycemics—insulin may or may not be needed. Children with type 2 diabetes who are overweight should be encouraged to lose weight.

ANIMATION

Responding to Hypoglycemia

VIDEO CLIPS

Adolescent Diabetes and Quality of Life

SUGGESTIONS FOR CLASSROOM ACTIVITIES

- Before class, assign students to complete "Case Study: Child with Type 1 Diabetes Returning to Elementary School," available on *mynursingkit .com*. Use this case study as a framework for discussing the transition from the acute care setting to the home environment.
- Ask the class which is more dangerous for a child with type 1 diabetes: hypoglycemia or hyperglycemia. Discuss the differences between the two conditions and the acute treatment of each.

SUGGESTIONS FOR CLINICAL ACTIVITIES

- Assign students to observe in an outpatient clinic that follows children with diabetes. Students can then compare and contrast these two different disease processes.
- When caring for a child with diabetes, review the age-appropriate signs and symptoms of hypoglycemia with the student. Discuss how hypoglycemia might be treated with that particular child.

LEARNING OUTCOME 7

Develop a nursing care plan for the child with an inherited metabolic disorder.

Concepts for Lecture

1. Children with inherited metabolic disorders often require special diets to manage their condition. Medication may be administered in some conditions (such as congenital hypothyroidism). Parents often need support and encouragement.

POWERPOINT SLIDES 56–58

SUGGESTION FOR CLASSROOM ACTIVITIES

- Before class, assign students to complete the activity "Thinking Critically: Child with Inborn Errors of Metabolism," available on *mynursingkit.com*. Use this activity as a framework to discuss this outcome in class.

SUGGESTION FOR CLINICAL ACTIVITIES

- Invite a dietitian to speak with the students during a clinical conference regarding the various formulas and dietary modifications required for children with congenital metabolic disorders.

GENERAL CHAPTER CONSIDERATIONS

1. Have students study and learn key terms listed at beginning of chapter.
2. Have students complete end-of-chapter exercises either in their book or on the MyNursingKit website.
3. Use the Classroom Response Questions provided in PowerPoint to assess students prior to lecture.

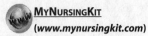

(www.mynursingkit.com)

- NCLEX RN® review questions
- Case Studies
- Care Plans
- Critical Concept Review
- Thinking Critically
- Weblinks
- Weblink applications
- Nursing Tools
- Audio Glossary
- Images and Tables Library

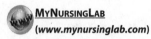

(www.mynursinglab.com)

- Knowledge Quick Check
- Pre/Posttests
- Customized study plans
- Images and Tables Library
- *Separate purchase*

CLINICAL SKILLS MANUAL

- *Separate purchase*

PEARSON eTEXT

- Students can search, highlight, take notes, and more all in electronic format
- *Separate purchase*

TESTBANK

CHAPTER 56
THE CHILD WITH ALTERATIONS IN NEUROLOGIC FUNCTION

LEARNING OUTCOME 1

Describe the anatomy and physiology of the neurologic system.

Concepts for Lecture

1. The basic structures of the neurologic system are the brain, spinal cord, and the nerves. Due to anatomic differences, children are at risk for different injuries to the central nervous system than adults.
2. The nervous system is immature at birth, and continues to develop during the first 4 years of life.

 POWERPOINT SLIDES 20–24

Figure 56–1. Transverse section of the brain and spinal cord

Feature Box: As Children Grow: Anatomic Differences between Children's and Adults' Nervous System Structures

 ANIMATION

3-D Brain and Brainstem

 SUGGESTION FOR CLASSROOM ACTIVITIES

- While discussing the anatomy of the nervous system, use the animation "3-D Brain and Brainstem," available on *mynursingkit.com*

 SUGGESTION FOR CLINICAL ACTIVITIES

- While in the clinical setting, locate CT scans of the head. Identify anatomic structures that are visible on the CT scans.

LEARNING OUTCOME 2

Describe the nursing assessment process and tools used for infants and children with altered levels of consciousness and other neurologic conditions.

Concepts for Lecture

1. Level of consciousness (LOC) is one of the most important indicators of neurologic dysfunction. It is important to understand the differences in the terms used to describe LOC.
2. Decline of a child's LOC follows a sequential pattern of deterioration. Close assessment and monitoring helps detect changes in the child's status. The Glasgow Coma Scale (GCS) is a tool that aims to quantify the child's LOC.

 POWERPOINT SLIDES 25–34

Table 56–2. Glasgow Coma Scale for assessment of coma in infants and children

 SUGGESTION FOR CLASSROOM ACTIVITIES

- Have a student volunteer to act out the changes that a child goes through as LOC decreases.

 SUGGESTION FOR CLINICAL ACTIVITIES

- Have students practice assessing LOC using the Glasgow Coma Scale on children of various ages.

LEARNING OUTCOME 3

Differentiate between the signs of infants and children with epilepsy and status epilepticus, and describe appropriate nursing management for each condition.

 POWERPOINT SLIDES 35–45

Feature Box: Clinical Manifestations: Seizures

Concepts for Lecture

1. Children may have a wide variety of seizures, although the most common type is tonic-clonic seizures. Refer to "Clinical Manifestations: Seizures" for details.
2. The main distinguishing factor between epilepsy and status epilepticus is the length of the seizure.
3. The basic nursing interventions for epilepsy and status epilepticus are similar and are focused on stopping the seizure and keeping the child safe. Children with status epilepticus will require more aggressive measures to stop their seizures, and may need airway management as well.

LEARNING OUTCOME 4

Differentiate between signs of bacterial meningitis, viral meningitis, encephalitis, and Guillain-Barré syndrome in infants and children.

Concepts for Lecture

1. Bacterial meningitis is characterized by fever, lethargy, vomiting, headache, and nuchal rigidity. Children with meningococcal meningitis also have a hemorrhagic rash.
2. The symptoms of viral meningitis are similar to those of bacterial meningitis. Viral meningitis is less severe than bacterial meningitis, and symptoms tend to be less intense.
3. Encephalitis is an inflammation of the brain, usually caused by a viral infection. Meningeal irritation may be present in addition to a wide variety of neurologic symptoms.
4. Guillain-Barré syndrome is characterized by deteriorating motor function and paralysis that progresses in an ascending pattern.

Feature Box: Drug Guide: Medications Used to Treat Seizures

ANIMATION

Diazepam

VIDEO CLIPS

Seizure Disorders

SUGGESTIONS FOR CLASSROOM ACTIVITIES

- To introduce the topic of seizures, show the video "Seizure Disorders," available on *mynursingkit.com*, at the beginning of this outcome.
- Show the animation "Diazepam" available on *mynursingkit.com*

SUGGESTION FOR CLINICAL ACTIVITIES

- When students are caring for children with seizure disorders, discuss the concept of "seizure precautions," as well as the rationale for the required equipment that is at the child's bedside. Review initial interventions the student should begin if the child has a seizure.

POWERPOINT SLIDES 46–67

Figure 56–5. Bacterial meningitis

Figure 56–6. Testing for Kernig and Brudzinski signs

SUGGESTION FOR CLASSROOM ACTIVITIES

- To help students differentiate between these disease processes, create case studies of children that display the common signs and symptoms of each disease process and have students determine which disease the child has based on the signs and symptoms you describe.

SUGGESTION FOR CLINICAL ACTIVITIES

- Lumbar punctures are commonly used with these disorders as a part of the diagnostic workup. Review the nurse's role in assisting with the lumbar puncture and discuss positioning of the child after the procedure is completed. If possible, have students assist with lumbar punctures.

LEARNING OUTCOME 5

Develop a nursing care plan for the infant with myelodysplasia and hydrocephalus.

Concepts for Lecture

1. Pre-op nursing care for children with myelodysplasia is focused on protecting the meningocele, while post-op care is focused on monitoring for signs of infection, hydrocephalus, and increased intracranial pressure.
2. Nursing care for the child with hydrocephalus includes positioning, and monitoring for signs of shunt malfunction, infection, and increased intracranial pressure.

POWERPOINT SLIDES 68–73

VIDEO CLIPS

Living with Spina Bifida

SUGGESTION FOR CLASSROOM ACTIVITIES

• At the beginning of this outcome, show the video "Living with Spina Bifida," available on *mynursingkit.com,* as a way to introduce this disorder.

SUGGESTION FOR CLINICAL ACTIVITIES

• Assign students to observe in the operating room to observe a myelomeningocele repair or a shunt insertion/revision.

LEARNING OUTCOME 6

Describe the focus of community-based nursing care for the child with cerebral palsy.

Concepts for Lecture

1. Cerebral palsy is commonly caused by injury to the central nervous system. Very premature infants are at high risk for developing cerebral palsy.
2. Nurses in the community play a critical role in coordinating care for the child with cerebral palsy.

POWERPOINT SLIDES 74–77

SUGGESTION FOR CLASSROOM ACTIVITIES

• Invite a family who has a child with cerebral palsy to speak to the class about how nurses can provide optimal care for these children in the community setting.

SUGGESTION FOR CLINICAL ACTIVITIES

• If there are facilities that care for children with cerebral palsy in the community, assign students to observe nurses working in the facility.

LEARNING OUTCOME 7

Distinguish among the assessment findings of the child with a mild, moderate, and severe traumatic brain injury.

Concepts for Lecture

1. Brain injury can be classified into three categories: mild, moderate, and severe. Assessment findings differ among these three groups. "Clinical Manifestations: Traumatic Brain Injury by Severity" is the primary reference for this outcome.

POWERPOINT SLIDES 78–83

Feature Box: Clinical Manifestations: Traumatic Brain Injury by Severity

ANIMATION

Coup-Contrecoup Injury

SUGGESTION FOR CLASSROOM ACTIVITIES

• The signs and symptoms of brain injury are directly related to the mechanism of injury. To illustrate this concept, use the animation "Coup-Contrecoup Injury," available on *mynursingkit.com*

SUGGESTION FOR CLINICAL ACTIVITIES

• Visit the radiology department to locate CT scans of children with head injuries of varying severity. What radiographic abnormalities are present in each type of head injury?

LEARNING OUTCOME 8

Contrast the appropriate initial nursing management for mild and severe traumatic brain injury.

Concepts for Lecture

1. Nursing management of mild brain injury involves monitoring level of consciousness and instructing parents on home monitoring parameters.
2. Nursing management of severe brain injury includes stabilization of vital signs, frequent monitoring, administering medications, and supporting the family.

GENERAL CHAPTER CONSIDERATIONS

1. Have students study and learn key terms listed at beginning of chapter.
2. Have students complete end-of-chapter exercises either in their book or on the MyNursingKit website.
3. Use the Classroom Response Questions provided in PowerPoint to assess students prior to lecture.

 POWERPOINT SLIDES 84–89

 SUGGESTION FOR CLASSROOM ACTIVITIES

- Before class, assign students to complete the exercise "Thinking Critically: Traumatic Brain Injury Death Prevention," available on *mynursingkit.com*. Use this activity to frame the discussion about prevention of brain injuries. Assign "Case Study: Post-Concussion Return to Competitive Play" activity on *mynursingkit.com* for homework.

 SUGGESTION FOR CLINICAL ACTIVITIES

- Assign students to observe or care for clients in the pediatric ICU, where many children with severe brain injury are cared for. In addition, consider assigning students to a pediatric rehabilitation hospital in order to see the long-term care required for many of these children.

 MYNURSINGKIT
(www.mynursingkit.com)

- NCLEX RN® review questions
- Case Studies
- Care Plans
- Critical Concept Review
- Thinking Critically
- Weblinks
- Weblink applications
- Nursing Tools
- Audio Glossary
- Images and Tables Library

 MYNURSINGLAB
(www.mynursinglab.com)

- Knowledge Quick Check
- Pre/Posttests
- Customized study plans
- Images and Tables Library
- *Separate purchase*

CLINICAL SKILLS MANUAL

- *Separate purchase*

 PEARSON ETEXT

- Students can search, highlight, take notes, and more all in electronic format
- *Separate purchase*

 TESTBANK

Chapter 57
The Child with Alterations in Mental Health and Cognitive Function

Learning Outcome 1

Define mental health and describe major mental health alterations in childhood.

Concepts for Lecture

1. Mental health is foundational to a sense of personal well-being. It involves the successful engagement in activities and relationships and the ability to adapt to and cope with change.
2. The major mental health alterations in childhood include pervasive developmental disorders, attention deficit and attention deficit hyperactivity disorder, mood disorders, anxiety disorders, tic disorders, and schizophrenia.

 PowerPoint Slides 20–29

 Video Clips

ADD/ADHD

 Suggestion for Classroom Activities

- Show the video "ADD/ADHD," located on *mynursingkit.com* as an introduction to the topic.

 Suggestion for Clinical Activities

- Assign students to observe in the mental health or psychiatric unit of the hospital to observe pediatric patients with these disease processes.

Learning Outcome 2

Discuss the clinical manifestations of the major mental health alterations of childhood and adolescence.

Concepts for Lecture

1. The clinical manifestations of major mental health disorders of childhood vary by disease. Most of these disorders have a range of symptoms from mild to severe.

 PowerPoint Slides 30–36

 Suggestion for Classroom Activities

- Act out the clinical manifestations of various mental health conditions, and see if the class can determine which disorder you are depicting. Then, discuss the clinical manifestations in more detail.

 Suggestion for Clinical Activities

- Students often find it helpful for the instructor to review terms used to describe mental health conditions objectively in the clinical setting.

Learning Outcome 3

Plan for nursing management of children and adolescents with mental health alterations in the hospital and community settings.

Concepts for Lecture

1. Overarching nursing management principles can be applied in the management of children with mental health disorders in both the hospital and the community.

 PowerPoint Slides 37–44

2. Each mental health alteration has a unique set of nursing interventions that is helpful in working with children with that alteration.

SUGGESTION FOR CLASSROOM ACTIVITIES

- Many families seek out health information on the Internet; however, information on websites may or may not be accurate. To encourage students to think about this issue, assign them to research any mental health disorder on the Internet and evaluate the information they find as to whether it is reliable or questionable. Discuss how the nurse can help families to evaluate mental health information on the Internet. Use some of the links provided in the Weblinks section located on *mynursingkit.com*

SUGGESTION FOR CLINICAL ACTIVITIES

- Have students attend an outpatient support group for children and families with the disorders described previously in this chapter.

LEARNING OUTCOME 4

Describe characteristics of common cognitive alterations of childhood.

Concepts for Lecture

1. Cognitive disorders can range from behaviors displayed in school to physical signs that are visible at birth. There is a wide array of cognitive disorders ranging from mild to severe. The text focuses on learning disabilities and intellectual disabilities (mental retardation).
2. Learning disabilities are a common problem in childhood, affecting about 5% of school children. The brain cannot receive or process information in the normal manner, causing difficulty in areas such as reading, writing, math, or understanding oral information. The child's IQ is usually normal.
3. Intellectual disability is now the preferred term for what was previously called mental retardation. Intellectual disability is a significant limitation in intellectual functioning and adaptive behavior. It begins in childhood, and the IQ is usually less than 70 to 75. Common syndromes associated with mental retardation include Down syndrome, fragile X syndrome, and fetal alcohol syndrome. Intellectual disabilities can also be associated with external or biologic factors.

POWERPOINT SLIDES 45–56

VIDEO CLIPS

Down Syndrome

SUGGESTION FOR CLASSROOM ACTIVITIES

- Show the video "Down Syndrome," available on *mynursingkit.com,* to illustrate the characteristics of this syndrome during the lecture.

SUGGESTION FOR CLINICAL ACTIVITIES

- When caring for children with one of the syndromes that is associated with mental retardation, have students practice the concept of the "functional assessment" described previously.

LEARNING OUTCOME 5

Plan nursing management for children with cognitive alterations.

Concepts for Lecture

1. Nursing management for children with intellectual disability focuses on early screening and detection, referral to intervention and support programs, and partnering with parents during hospitalization.
2. Nursing management for children with learning disabilities focuses on early detection, referral, goal setting, and promotion of self-esteem.

POWERPOINT SLIDES 57–62

Feature Box: Evidence-Based Nursing: Family Needs During Hospitalization for Mental Health Care.

SUGGESTION FOR CLASSROOM ACTIVITIES

- Have the class take a few minutes to read "Evidence-Based Nursing: Family Needs During Hospitalization for Mental Health Care." Use the critical thinking questions at the end to discuss the needs families express during hospitalization. How might these needs differ from families of children with chronic illness (e.g., the family with a child who has an intellectual disability)?

SUGGESTION FOR CLINICAL ACTIVITIES

- Discuss practical strategies students can use to negotiate hospital care routines with the family of a child who is mentally retarded. Discuss the benefits to partnering with the family in this situation.

LEARNING OUTCOME 6

Establish and evaluate expected outcomes of care for the child with a cognitive alteration.

Concepts for Lecture

1. The expected outcomes of nursing care depend on the child's needs and developmental level.
2. Early outcomes focus on the understanding of the diagnosis, while later outcomes focus on the child's skills, as well as utilization of resources in the community.

POWERPOINT SLIDES 63–65

SUGGESTION FOR CLASSROOM ACTIVITIES

- Ask the class how they would evaluate the outcomes described in this outcome. Discuss as a group the nursing evaluation of a child in the school with a cognitive disorder. What can be done to enhance the achievement of these goals by the nurse? What community organizations are available to help?

SUGGESTION FOR CLINICAL ACTIVITIES

- Have students identify local resources in their community that might be helpful for families who have children with mental retardation.

GENERAL CHAPTER CONSIDERATIONS

1. Have students study and learn key terms listed at beginning of chapter.
2. Have students complete end of chapter exercises either in their book or on the MyNursingKit website.
3. Use the Classroom Response Questions provided in PowerPoint to assess students prior to lecture.

MYNURSINGKIT
(*www.mynursingkit.com*)

- NCLEX RN® review questions
- Case Studies
- Care Plans
- Critical Concept Review
- Thinking Critically
- Weblinks
- Weblink applications
- Nursing Tools
- Audio Glossary
- Images and Tables Library

MYNURSINGLAB
(*www.mynursinglab.com*)

- Knowledge Quick Check
- Pre/Posttests
- Customized study plans
- Images and Tables Library
- *Separate purchase*

CLINICAL SKILLS MANUAL

- *Separate purchase*

PEARSON ETEXT

- Students can search, highlight, take notes, and more all in electronic format
- *Separate purchase*

TESTBANK

CHAPTER 58
THE CHILD WITH ALTERATIONS IN MUSCULOSKELETAL FUNCTION

LEARNING OUTCOME 1

Describe pediatric variations in the musculoskeletal system.

Concepts for Lecture

1. The skeletal system continues to grow and mature throughout childhood. Growth takes place at the epiphyseal plates, which are located near the ends of the bones. In addition, the bones of children are porous and less dense than those of adults, making them more likely to bend, buckle, and break. However, bones tend to heal quickly due to rapid bone growth.
2. Unlike the skeletal system, the muscular system is almost completely formed at birth. Muscles increase in length and circumference but not in number. Until puberty, both ligaments and tendons are stronger than bone. As a result, fractures are sometimes mistaken for sprains.

LEARNING OUTCOME 2

Plan nursing care for children with structural deformities of the foot, hip, and spine.

Concepts for Lecture

1. Structural disorders of the feet and legs include metatarsus adductus, clubfoot, genu varum, and genu valgum.
2. Structural disorders of the hip include hip dysplasia, Legg-Calvé-Perthes disease, and slipped capital femoral epiphysis.
3. Structural disorders of the spine include scoliosis, torticollis, kyphosis, and lordosis.

 POWERPOINT SLIDES 20–26

Figure 58–2. The parts of long bones

 ANIMATION

Muscle Physiology

 SUGGESTION FOR CLASSROOM ACTIVITIES

- Use the animation "Muscle Physiology," available on *mynursingkit.com,* to review how muscles work. This concept is important in order to understand disease processes that affect the musculoskeletal system.

 SUGGESTION FOR CLINICAL ACTIVITIES

- Examine x-rays of children of different ages. Look for the differences in bone size, as well as the epiphyseal plate.

 POWERPOINT SLIDES 27–57

Figure 58–3. Metatarsus adductus

Figure 58–5. Genu valgum and genu varum

Figure 58–6. Common signs of developmental dysplasia of the hip (DDH)

Figure 58–7. Pavlik harness for DDH

Figure 58–8. Spica cast

Figure 58–9. Toronto brace

Figure 58–10. Clues for early detection of scoliosis

Feature Box: Pathophysiology Illustrated: Clubfoot

Feature Box: Pathophysiology Illustrated: Slipped Epiphysis

- Due to the high incidence of scoliosis in girls, it is common for several students in a class to have scoliosis. Ask the class if anyone is willing to share how the condition is monitored and treated.

SUGGESTION FOR CLINICAL ACTIVITIES

- Have students screen adolescent clients for scoliosis.

LEARNING OUTCOME 3

Recognize signs and symptoms of infectious musculoskeletal disorders and refer for appropriate care.

Concepts for Lecture

1. Osteomyelitis is an infection of the bone that may be acute or chronic, and treatment involves antimicrobial therapy.
2. Skeletal tuberculosis and septic arthritis occur infrequently in children. Refer to "Clinical Manifestations: Skeletal Tuberculosis and Septic Arthritis" for a summary.

POWERPOINT SLIDES 58–63

Feature Box: Clinical Manifestations: Skeletal Tuberculosis and Septic Arthritis

SUGGESTION FOR CLASSROOM ACTIVITIES

- Discuss why long-term IV antibiotics are required to treat infections involving bones and joints. What makes these infections different from a lung or ear infection?

SUGGESTION FOR CLINICAL ACTIVITIES

- If a child will require long-term home IV antimicrobial therapy, have students identify local resources available in their community to achieve this therapy. For example, are parents taught to administer the antibiotics themselves, or do nurses make home visits? What kinds of long-term IV access are available, and what are the risks of these devices?

LEARNING OUTCOME 4

Partner with families to plan care for children with musculoskeletal conditions that are chronic or require long-term care.

Concepts for Lecture

1. Achondroplasia (dwarfism) is a genetic condition where the head and torso are normal, but the arms and legs are short in size. There is no treatment for this disorder so nursing care focuses on helping families develop a positive self-image for the child.
2. Marfan syndrome is a genetic condition that involves the connective tissue. There are cardiac, skeletal, and respiratory manifestations of the disease. Although there are no specific treatments, surgery may be done to prevent dissection of the aorta, which is the major cause of death.
3. Osteogenesis imperfecta, also known as brittle bone disease, is a collagen disorder. These children have frequent fractures, as well as other physical symptoms. Management is focused on preventing fractures and deformities.
4. Muscular dystrophy refers to a group of inherited diseases characterized by muscle fiber degeneration and muscle wasting. They are all terminal disorders, although the progression varies from a few years to

POWERPOINT SLIDES 64–75

SUGGESTION FOR CLASSROOM ACTIVITIES

- It is likely that both Abraham Lincoln and Jonathan Larson (composer of the musical *Rent*) had Marfan syndrome. Show pictures of Lincoln and Larson when discussing the physical manifestations of the disease process. Larson died from a ruptured aortic aneurysm shortly before *Rent* premiered, so students may use this fact to remember the most serious complication of the disease.

SUGGESTION FOR CLINICAL ACTIVITIES

- During clinical conference, discuss possible complications of muscular dystrophy that may require children to be admitted to the hospital. Discuss how the nurse can offer psychosocial support to these children and families.

many years. Nursing care focuses on the parent and the child, and includes promoting independence and mobility, emotional support, and acceptance of the disease process.

LEARNING OUTCOME 5

Plan nursing interventions to promote safety and developmental progression in children who require braces, casts, traction, and surgery.

Concepts for Lecture

1. Nursing care of children who require braces, casts, traction, and surgery varies by age. Resources available in the text include Tables 58-1 and 58-4, as well as "Teaching Highlights: Care of the Child with a Cast" and "Teaching Highlights: Guidelines for Brace Wear."

 POWERPOINT SLIDES 76–80

Table 58–1. Nursing care of the child in a cast

Table 58–4. Care of the child with traction or external fixator

Feature Box: Teaching Highlights: Care of the Child with a Cast

Feature Box: Teaching Highlights: Guidelines for Brace Wear

Feature Box: Clinical Manifestations: Compartment Syndrome

 SUGGESTION FOR CLASSROOM ACTIVITIES

• In class, review Table 58-1, Nursing Care of the Child in a Cast. Use this as a basis to discuss developmental considerations for children requiring casts.

 SUGGESTION FOR CLINICAL ACTIVITIES

• Review the signs and symptoms of compartment syndrome when discussing care of the child in a cast. If a child is displaying these signs and symptoms, discuss the appropriate actions the nurse should take. "Clinical Manifestations: Compartment Syndrome" is a good resource.

LEARNING OUTCOME 6

Provide nursing care for fractures, including teaching for injury prevention and nursing implementations for the child who has sustained a fracture.

Concepts for Lecture

1. Fractures can occur at any age, and may result from direct trauma to bones or from diseases that weaken the bone. Refer to "Pathophysiology Illustrated: Classification and Types of Fractures" for details regarding types of fractures. Nursing care focuses on maintaining proper alignment, monitoring neurovascular status, pain control, and discharge teaching.
2. Sports injuries are a common cause of fractures in children. Refer to Table 58-5. Many sports injuries can be prevented.

 POWERPOINT SLIDES 81–86

Table 58–5. Common sports injuries

Feature Box: Pathophysiology Illustrated: Classification and Types of Fractures

 SUGGESTION FOR CLASSROOM ACTIVITIES

• Before class, assign students to access "Case Study: Fracture Assessment" located on *mynursingkit.com*. Use this as a basis for discussion regarding management of fractures during childhood.

 SUGGESTION FOR CLINICAL ACTIVITIES

• Demonstrate methods to assess neurovascular status in infants and toddlers. How do these methods vary from older children?

General Chapter Considerations

1. Have students study and learn key terms listed at beginning of chapter.
2. Have students complete end-of-chapter exercises either in their book or on the MyNursingKit website.
3. Use the Classroom Response Questions provided in PowerPoint to assess students prior to lecture.

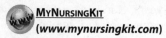

MyNursingKit (*www.mynursingkit.com*)

- NCLEX RN® review questions
- Case Studies
- Care Plans
- Critical Concept Review
- Thinking Critically
- Weblinks
- Weblink applications
- Nursing Tools
- Audio Glossary
- Images and Tables Library

MyNursingLab (*www.mynursinglab.com*)

- Knowledge Quick Check
- Pre/Posttests
- Customized study plans
- Images and Tables Library
- *Separate purchase*

Clinical Skills Manual

- *Separate purchase*

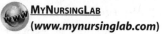

Pearson eText

- Students can search, highlight, take notes, and more all in electronic format
- *Separate purchase*

Testbank

CHAPTER 59
THE CHILD WITH ALTERATIONS IN SKIN INTEGRITY

LEARNING OUTCOME 1

Identify the characteristics of different skin lesions by their cause, including those caused by irritants, drug reactions, mites, infection, and injury.

Concepts for Lecture

1. The characteristics of skin lesions vary based on their cause.

LEARNING OUTCOME 2

Describe the stages of wound healing.

Concepts for Lecture

1. There are three distinct stages in wound healing: inflammation, reconstruction (or proliferation), and maturation (or remodeling). Refer to "Pathophysiology Illustrated: Phases of Wound Healing" for graphic representations of these stages.

 POWERPOINT SLIDES 15–20

 SUGGESTIONS FOR CLASSROOM ACTIVITIES

- Divide students into groups and provide each group with a set of colored pencils and a blank piece of paper. Have each group draw one of the lesions described previously, including the common characteristics of that lesion. Share each group's drawing with the class.
- Before class, have the students do the Weblink Application "Head Lice," available on *mynursingkit.com*. Use this as a basis for discussion of infestation control in schools.

 SUGGESTION FOR CLINICAL ACTIVITIES

- When a student is caring for a child with a skin lesion, review the proper terminology used for documentation. Students often have difficulty describing what they are seeing.

 POWERPOINT SLIDES 21–25

Feature Box: Pathophysiology Illustrated: Phases of Wound Healing

 ANIMATION:

Integumentary Repair

Activity: Layers of the Skin

 SUGGESTIONS FOR CLASSROOM ACTIVITIES

- Use the animation "Integumentary Repair" located on *mynursingkit.com* to give students a visual representation of this process during the lecture.
- Have students do the activity: Layers of the Skin located on *mynursingkit.com* for homework.

SUGGESTION FOR CLINICAL ACTIVITIES

- Have students discuss how the stage of wound healing their client is in impacts their nursing care.

LEARNING OUTCOME 3

Describe a nursing care plan for a child with acute skin disorders, including dermatitis, infectious disorders, and infestations.

Concepts for Lecture

1. The nursing model can be applied to create a nursing care plan for the child with acute skin disorders, including assessment, diagnosis, planning and implementation, and evaluation.

LEARNING OUTCOME 4

Plan the nursing care for the child with a chronic skin condition.

Concepts for Lecture

1. Atopic eczema (also known as atopic dermatitis) is a chronic, relapsing, superficial inflammatory skin disorder characterized by intense pruritus. It affects infants, children, and adolescents. Those who will have the disorder usually develop it early in life. Eczema is characterized by red patches with exudates and crust.

LEARNING OUTCOME 5

Develop an education plan for adolescents with acne to promote self-care.

Concepts for Lecture

1. Acne is a chronic inflammatory disorder that is the most common skin disorder in the pediatric population.
2. Clinical therapies for acne include topical keratolytics, topical antibiotics, topical retinoids, oral antibiotics, and oral isotretinoin.
3. Education for the adolescent with acne focuses on triggers of acne, skin cleansing routines, medications, and side effects. Psychologic support should also be considered. Refer to "Nursing Care Plan: The Adolescent with Acne."

 POWERPOINT SLIDES 26–30

 SUGGESTION FOR CLASSROOM ACTIVITIES

- Before class, assign students to read about acute skin conditions. During class, have them apply their knowledge to create a nursing care plan for a child with an acute skin condition.

 SUGGESTION FOR CLINICAL ACTIVITIES

- Consider assigning students to an outpatient dermatology office that treats pediatric clients. Have the student evaluate the nursing care provided during the visit.

 POWERPOINT SLIDES 31–36

Figure 59–7. Chronic eczema

 SUGGESTION FOR CLASSROOM ACTIVITIES

- Before class, assign students to review the "Care Plan: Atopic Dermatitis," located on *mynursingkit.com*. Use this care plan as a basis for discussing the disease process.

 SUGGESTION FOR CLINICAL ACTIVITIES

- When students are caring for a child with eczema, review the importance of applying ointments right after bathing in order to trap moisture in the skin.

 POWERPOINT SLIDES 37–42

Feature Box: Nursing Care Plan: The Adolescent with Acne

 SUGGESTION FOR CLASSROOM ACTIVITIES

- Before class, assign students to read Nursing Care Plan: The Adolescent with Acne. Use this as a basis for discussing this outcome.

 SUGGESTION FOR CLINICAL ACTIVITIES

- Discuss typical topical and systemic medications used to treat acne, as well as the precautions that must be followed while adolescents take these medications.

LEARNING OUTCOME 6

Describe the process to measure the extent of burns and burn severity in children.

Concepts for Lecture

1. Burns are a common type of injury in pediatrics. There are four types of burns, including thermal, chemical, electrical, and radioactive. Children are at risk for different types of burns based on their developmental age.
2. Burns are classified by their depth, percentage of body surface area affected, and the involvement of specific body parts. Refer to "Pathophysiology Illustrated: Classification of Burns by Depth."

LEARNING OUTCOME 7

Develop a nursing care plan for the child with a full-thickness burn injury.

Concepts for Lecture

1. Assessment of the child with full thickness burns includes airway assessment, breathing, and circulation; history and type of burn; possibility of other injuries; pain assessment, and close attention to fluid status. The burn should be consistent with the history, as about 10–25% of burns in children are due to child abuse.
2. Diagnosis helps guide nursing interventions. Refer to "Nursing Care Plan: The Child with a Major Burn Injury" for detailed interventions.
3. Evaluation is done to determine the effectiveness of nursing interventions.

LEARNING OUTCOME 8

Identify preventive strategies to reduce the risk of injury from burns, hypothermia, bites and stings.

Concepts for Lecture

1. There are numerous prevention strategies to prevent bites and stings from insects.
2. Burn prevention should be discussed at health promotion visits.

 POWERPOINT SLIDES 43–49

Figure 59–13. Lund and Browder chart with BSA distributions

Feature Box: Pathophysiology Illustrated: Classification of Burns by Depth

 SUGGESTION FOR CLINICAL ACTIVITIES

- Using scenarios that you create, have students practice using the Lund and Browder chart to determine the percentage of a child's body that has been burned.

 POWERPOINT SLIDES 50–56

Figure 59–15. Burn injuries associated with child abuse

Feature Box: Nursing Care Plan: The Child with a Major Burn Injury

 VIDEO CLIPS

Nursing in Action: Topical Medication: Burn Wound Care

 SUGGESTION FOR CLASSROOM ACTIVITIES

- Before class, assign students to complete the "Nursing in Action: Topical Medication: Burn Wound Care" activity, located on *mynursingkit.com*. Use this as a framework for discussion about nursing care of the child with a major burn.

 SUGGESTION FOR CLINICAL ACTIVITIES

- Assign students to observe in a burn unit. If a burn unit is not available in your clinical setting, see if the physical therapy department treats burn clients on an outpatient basis and assign students to observe those treatments.

 POWERPOINT SLIDES 57–61

 SUGGESTION FOR CLASSROOM ACTIVITIES

- If you would like to have students think about prevention of dog bites, assign them to complete "Thinking Critically: Develop a Community Education Program: Dog Bite Reduction," located on *mynursingkit.com*

3. Hypothermia can be prevented when exposure to cold temperatures is likely.

GENERAL CHAPTER CONSIDERATIONS

1. Have students study and learn key terms listed at beginning of chapter.
2. Have students complete end of chapter exercises either in their book or on the MyNursingKit website.
3. Use the Classroom Response Questions provided in PowerPoint to assess students prior to lecture.

 SUGGESTION FOR CLINICAL ACTIVITIES

- Consider discussing the following questions while in the clinical setting: What are some of the serious clinical consequences of bites and stings? What diseases can be transmitted by insects? How can prevention strategies be communicated to parents?

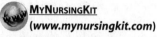 **MYNURSINGKIT**
(www.mynursingkit.com)

- NCLEX RN® review questions
- Case Studies
- Care Plans
- Critical Concept Review
- Thinking Critically
- Weblinks
- Weblink applications
- Nursing Tools
- Audio Glossary
- Images and Tables Library

 MYNURSINGLAB
(www.mynursinglab.com)

- Knowledge Quick Check
- Pre/Posttests
- Customized study plans
- Images and Tables Library
- *Separate purchase*

CLINICAL SKILLS MANUAL

- *Separate purchase*

 PEARSON eTEXT

- Students can search, highlight, take notes, and more all in electronic format
- *Separate purchase*

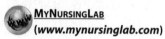 **TESTBANK**